The
Fertility Diet

Groundbreaking Research Reveals Natural Ways to Boost

Ovulation & Improve Your Chances of Getting Pregnant

JORGE E. CHAVARRO, M.D., Sc.D.

WALTER C. WILLETT, M.D., Dr.P.H.

PATRICK J. SKERRETT

Mc Graw Hill

New York Chicago San Francisco Lisbon London Madrid Mexico City
Milan New Delhi San Juan Seoul Singapore Sydney Toronto

8 9 10 11 12 13 14 15 16   QFR/QFR   1 9 8 7 6 5

ISBN 978-0-07-162710-8
MHID   0-07-162710-3

Library of Congress Cataloging-in-Publication Data

Chavarro, Jorge.
        The fertility diet / by Jorge Chavarro, Walter C. Willett, and Patrick J. Skerrett.
            p.   cm.
        Includes bibliographical references and index.
        ISBN 978-0-07-162710-8 (alk. paper)
        MHID 0-07-162710-3 (alk. paper)
        1. Infertility, Female—Diet therapy—Popular works.   2. Infertility, Female—
Diet therapy—Recipes.   3. Infertility, Female—Nutritional aspects—Popular
works.   I. Willett, Walter.   II. Skerrett, P. J. (Patrick J.), 1953–   III. Title.

        RG201.C43   2009
        618.1'780654—dc22   2008055591

Interior design by Susan H. Hartman
Figures 2.2 and 2.3 by Jennifer Fairman; Figures 2.4, 2.5, 2.7, 7.1, and 8.1 by Scott
Leighton; Figure 2.6 by Jesse Tarantino; Figure 3.1 by Christopher Bing; Figure 10.1 by Ed
Wiederer

Contents

Adopting any one of the ten steps the book recommends is a great start. Following more of them appears to be even better. Among the women in the Nurses' Health Study, those who followed five or more of the Fertility Diet strategies reduced their risk of ovulatory infertility by 80 percent to 90 percent. That's a substantial reduction achieved with a set of simple, inexpensive, and tasty dietary changes.

Throughout the book, Drs. Chavarro and Willett provide specific, practical advice about how to adjust your diet to improve fertility. A weeklong sample diet and recipes help translate this advice into practice. An additional bonus is that the diet they recommend is good for both a healthy pregnancy and a lifetime of healthy eating.

Other books have provided advice on diet and fertility. But none of them is based on the wealth of evidence provided by the Nurses' Health Study. And none of them comes from scientists with the stature of the authors of *The Fertility Diet*. Dr. Willett's contributions to the field of human nutrition have been so important that he is one of the most cited scientists in the world. The scientific publications by Drs. Chavarro and Willett and their colleagues on nutrition and fertility will undoubtedly bolster this impressive achievement and, more important, should lead the way to a new understanding of the sometimes obvious, sometimes subtle, connections between diet and reproduction.

A long list of problems can lead to infertility. A couple whose infertility stems from blocked fallopian tubes or low sperm production isn't likely to be helped by changes in diet and lifestyle. That's one reason why it makes sense to see a specialist if you are having trouble getting pregnant. That said, the two most common impediments to pregnancy are problems with ovulation and infertility for which no obvious cause can be found. For these, lifestyle changes that include an optimal diet, appropriate levels of exercise, reducing unnecessary stress, and eliminating exposure to nicotine can improve fertility.

A great paradox of modern medicine is that powerful and invasive high-tech approaches to infertility, such as in vitro fertilization, are widely available and highly effective for quickly achieving pregnancy. But they aren't the only solution. For many women who want to become pregnant, low-tech approaches such as optimizing diet and lifestyle

Foreword

██████████████████████

❝❝ Does my diet affect my chances of getting pregnant?"

That's a question I am asked all the time. Sometimes it comes from women grappling with infertility, other times from healthy women who are hoping to become pregnant. Although I have always answered in the affirmative, I haven't been able to base my answer on strong scientific evidence. Now I can.

Groundbreaking research from the Nurses' Health Study indicates that various components of diet, from fats to beverages, can help women avoid one of the most common causes of infertility—problems with ovulation, the carefully timed release of an egg from the ovary. This research, led by Drs. Jorge Chavarro and Walter Willett of the Harvard School of Public Health, lays the foundation for a dietary plan for fertility and beyond.

In *The Fertility Diet: Groundbreaking Research Reveals Natural Ways to Boost Ovulation and Improve Your Chances of Getting Pregnant,* Drs. Chavarro and Willett review the previously limited scientific evidence linking diet with fertility and present compelling findings on this connection from the Nurses' Health Study. They explain how (and why) "good" fats, whole grains, and plant protein help guard against ovulatory infertility, while "bad" fats, refined carbohydrates, and red meat may contribute to it. They make the case that full-fat dairy products seem to be good for fertility, while skim milk and sugared sodas aren't.

can significantly improve fertility and lead to pregnancy. Common sense suggests that this is the place to start. *The Fertility Diet* provides a map that guides couples toward diet and lifestyle choices that can make a real difference in fertility.

Robert L. Barbieri, M.D.
Chairman of Obstetrics, Gynecology, and Reproductive Biology, Brigham and Women's Hospital
Kate Macy Ladd Professor of Obstetrics, Gynecology, and Reproductive Biology, Harvard Medical School

Acknowledgments

I f many hands make light work, then the task of creating this book was featherlike. First and foremost, we would like to thank the participants of the Nurses' Health Study, especially the women in the fertility study. The information they have shared about their reproductive experiences, as well as about their diets and lifestyle choices, is the source of the new findings on diet and fertility described in this book. We also want to thank the members of the Nurses' Health Study research team, who routinely take mountains of seemingly random data and translate them into coherent pictures. In particular, we would like to acknowledge the special contributions of Janet Rich-Edwards, Sc.D., and Bernard Rosner, Ph.D., key members of the Nurses' Health Study research team, who helped us formulate many of the questions explored in our diet-fertility studies and then understand the answers.

We would be remiss if we did not acknowledge the support of the National Institutes of Health, which has provided important research funding for the Nurses' Healthy Study for many years. We very much appreciate the strong public support for health research in the United States and hope that the information in this book represents a good return on investment.

We also want to thank Robert Barbieri, M.D., chief of obstetrics, gynecology, and reproductive biology at Brigham and Women's Hospital, for reviewing the manuscript and ensuring that nutritional epidemiologists accurately presented the biology of reproduction, what can go wrong, and how nutrition may affect fertility.

We are indebted to our colleagues at Harvard Health Publications who helped take this book from idea to print. Editor-in-chief Anthony L. Komaroff, M.D.; chief editor for books Julie K. Silver, M.D.; and managing editor Nancy Ferrari provided valuable editorial guidance. Associate editor Raquel Schott kept us on track, especially in her coordination of figures and tables. Art director Heather Derocher and graphic design intern Merika Ficheux helped craft the illustrations that grace the book. At McGraw-Hill, editors Judith McCarthy and Julia Anderson Bauer smoothly ushered the book from conception to production.

Last, but never least, we want to thank our families:

Jorge Chavarro: I would like to thank my wife, Amy, for her support and encouragement throughout the research I did into possible links between diet and fertility. Who could have known that what began as a relatively small research project would grow into a book like this? I also want to acknowledge my daughter, Isabella, who was born during the writing of this book. I hope that the strategies described in *The Fertility Diet* will help many couples experience the kind of intense joy that Isabella has brought to our lives.

Walter Willett: I would like to thank my wife, Gail, for her support and tolerance of the many nights and weekends demanded by a research and writing career.

Pat Skerrett: I am forever grateful for the love, support, and encouragement that daily comes my way from my wife, Helen Dájer, and our children, Michael, Helen Claire, and Peter. Thanks for letting me take over the dining room table with infertility papers and for fighting my tunnel vision with baseball, dancing, and nighttime reading.

Chapter 1

Nourishing the Miracle of Conception

C onception, that frantic meeting between egg and sperm, is a fragile miracle. So many things must happen in just the right order
that it would seem to be improbable. Yet it happens all by itself
millions of times a year. For one in seven American couples, though,
conception doesn't "just happen."[1] Something thwarts the rendezvous
between sperm and egg. The list of these somethings is long, ranging from eggs that don't mature properly to blocked fallopian tubes
and weak-swimming sperm. Physical, physiological, and hormonal
barriers to conception mean baby making can take much longer than
expected or not happen at all.

Many couples keep trying, and hoping, and worrying. Others turn to
the burgeoning medical industry that has bloomed in the last couple
decades to get around barriers to conception. Medications that rev up
egg production along with an alphabet soup of reproductive procedures—IVF, GIFT, ZIFT, ICSI, and others—have helped more than a
million couples have babies.

These medical approaches aren't perfect. They lead to a viable
pregnancy only about one-quarter of the time. They are time consuming and invasive. They can have unwanted side effects. Many couples
would rather not turn to technology for something as intimate and personal as conceiving a child. Others simply can't afford it.

High-tech medicine isn't the only answer.

The Fertility Diet

Exciting new research from the Nurses' Health Study, one of the largest and longest-running studies of women's health in America, shows that what you eat, how active you are, and other lifestyle choices can stack the reproductive deck in your favor, especially if trouble with ovulation—the maturation or release of a mature egg each month—is at the root of your problems conceiving.

It is common knowledge that what you eat and how you live affect the health of your heart and blood vessels, your chances of developing certain kinds of cancer, your eyesight, the strength of your bones, and more. It only makes sense that diet and health affect the ability to get pregnant and stay pregnant. After all, reproduction is just one of many systems in the body, all of them subject to similar rules and influences.

What is astonishing is that this is news. While millions upon millions of dollars have been spent developing and perfecting reproductive technologies, almost no attention has been paid to connections between diet and fertility. This oversight speaks volumes about medicine in America—a laserlike focus on drugs, devices, or procedures that can generate revenue and often total disregard for self-help measures that anyone can do for free.

Ten Steps to Improving Your Fertility

Farmers, ranchers, and animal scientists know far more about how nutrition affects fertility in cows, pigs, sheep, chickens, and other commercially important animals than reproduction experts know about how it affects fertility in humans. To be sure, hints are scattered across medical journals. But there have been few systematic studies of this crucial connection in people.

We set out to change this sad state of affairs with the help of more than eighteen thousand female nurses from all across the United States. These women are part of the Nurses' Health Studies, which we describe in "Knowledge from Nurses." They have provided information

KNOWLEDGE FROM NURSES

More than thirty years ago, researchers hoping to answer a vitally important question—Do birth control pills have long-term health effects?—proposed a bold study. They would survey thousands of female nurses about their methods of birth control and then track their health over time. Little did they know that this study would evolve into one of the largest investigations of how diet, lifestyle, social, and biological factors affect the risk of developing heart disease, cancer, diabetes, osteoporosis, and other chronic conditions.

The researchers, from the Harvard School of Public Health, chose nurses for several reasons. Because of their knowledge and training, nurses could be counted on to provide accurate, reliable health information. Equally important, as health professionals, they are extremely aware of the value of medical research and have traditionally been willing to make long-term commitments to studies.

That commitment was evident from the get-go. The study started in 1976 with more than 120,000 married, female nurses between the ages of thirty and fifty-five. Each completed a two-page questionnaire. Every two years since then, these women have loyally filled out ever-expanding questionnaires asking about what they eat and how much they exercise, about work and stress, and about other personal matters such as social relationships and caregiving. They also provide detailed reports about the state of their health.

A second round of the Nurses' Health Study was started in 1989 by one of us (Dr. Willett) to explore reproductive and other health issues that couldn't be answered by the original study. It includes 116,000 younger women who also complete detailed questionnaires every other year.

This book is based on research conducted in a specially selected group of women from this second group. To help understand how diet affects fertility, we identified 18,555 participants who said on one of the biennial surveys that they were trying to get pregnant. None had previously reported problems with infertility. Over the next eight years, these women reported nearly 27,000 "pregnancy attempts." That doesn't mean 27,000 acts of intercourse (which would make this one of the most undersexed groups of women in America), but 27,000 efforts to get pregnant that lasted from a few weeks to more than twelve months. Most were successful. Slightly more than 3,400 of the women trying to have a baby (13 percent) had difficulty becoming pregnant, including hundreds who experienced ovulatory infertility.

Thanks to these women and the personal information they generously provided, we have been able to investigate connections between diet and fertility. We hope that the efforts of these dedicated nurses, which are embodied in this book, will help other women prevent or overcome ovulatory infertility.

You can learn more about the Nurses' Health Studies, and even see the questionnaires the participants complete, by visiting the study's website, www.nurseshealthstudy.org.

on their health, including pregnancies, miscarriages, and infertility, along with detailed records of their diets, physical activity, smoking habits, and other practices. All told, the women in the fertility study have contributed more than eighty million bits of data. From this vast mine of information, we have discovered ten simple changes that offer a powerful boost in fertility for women with ovulation-related infertility. These are:

1. Avoid trans fats, the artery-clogging fats found in many commercially prepared products and fast foods.
2. Use more unsaturated vegetable oils, such as olive oil or canola oil.
3. Eat more vegetable protein, like beans and nuts, and less animal protein.
4. Choose whole grains and other sources of carbohydrate that have lower, slower effects on blood sugar and insulin rather than highly refined carbohydrates that quickly boost blood sugar and insulin.
5. Drink a glass of whole milk or have a small dish of ice cream or full-fat yogurt every day; temporarily trade in skim milk and low- or no-fat dairy products like cottage cheese and frozen yogurt for their full-fat cousins.

6. Take a multivitamin that contains folic acid and other B vitamins.
7. Get plenty of iron from fruits, vegetables, beans, and supplements but not from red meat.
8. Beverages matter: water is great; coffee, tea, and alcohol are OK in moderation; stay away from sugared sodas.
9. Aim for a healthy weight. If you are overweight, losing between 5 and 10 percent of your weight can jump-start ovulation.
10. If you aren't physically active, start a daily exercise plan. If you already exercise, pick up the pace of your workouts. But don't overdo it, especially if you are quite lean—too much exercise can work against conception.

We didn't mention smoking. Only a small number of women in the Nurses' Health Study are smokers, which made it impossible for us to examine in detail its effects on fertility. We didn't really need to, though. Scads of solid studies have established that women who smoke take longer to get pregnant on their own or with assisted reproduction and are more likely to miscarry than nonsmokers.[2] So we'll add an eleventh recommendation: if you smoke, stop.

You may think that you've heard advice like this before. There are a few infertility diet books in circulation, and the Internet is rife with dietary advice for women who want to get pregnant. These are scatter-shot approaches based on wishful thinking and what seems like common sense. Our recommendations, on the other hand, are based on evidence from one of the most comprehensive long-term studies ever conducted.

At least for now, this advice is aimed at preventing and reversing ovulatory infertility. It may work for other types of infertility, but we don't yet have enough data to explore connections between nutrition and infertility due to other causes. Because the Nurses' Health Study doesn't include information on the participants' partners, we weren't able to explore whether nutrition affects male infertility. From what we have gleaned from the limited research in this area, though, some of the Fertility Diet strategies might improve fertility in men, too.

Good for All

These ten tips work on many levels. They are simple. They cost a few dollars at most. They don't have side effects, with the possible exception of twins, as we describe in "Double Take." They are available to everyone, not just those with good health insurance. Best of all, they are every bit as good for your long-term health—and your partner's—as they are for improving fertility. In fact, a diet built around these strategies will serve you well all through pregnancy and into old age.

DOUBLE TAKE

The ovaries are programmed to release one mature egg each cycle. Something goes awry with this process in up to one-quarter of couples who have trouble getting pregnant. Some women with ovulatory infertility have trouble making mature eggs. Others don't release them at the right time. One option is the use of fertility drugs such as clomiphene (Clomid) or injections of follicle-stimulating hormone or luteinizing hormone (Pergonal, Fertinex, and others) that ramp up the ovaries' production of eggs. The usual result of these drugs is the release of multiple mature eggs.

The changes we advise in the Fertility Diet improve ovulation, though in a less dramatic way. It is possible that even this gentler stimulation may prompt the ovaries to make and release more than one egg every so often. If both get fertilized, you could go from no children to two in a heartbeat.

As one of us (Skerrett) knows firsthand, twins can be a blessing. But they can also pose health risks to each other and their mother. Women carrying twins are more likely to develop gestational diabetes or preeclampsia than women carrying a single child. Twins tend to arrive earlier, with almost half of all twins born prematurely.[3] They can limit each other's growth, and fetal death is more common with twins.

Those are the possibilities. The reality is that most women carrying twins have safe, uneventful pregnancies and deliver two healthy children.

Using This Book

In the chapters that follow, we lay out how and why each of the ten steps affect fertility and offer tips for putting them into practice. Chapter 13 helps you plan a week's worth of meals and snacks and includes fifteen recipes that incorporate our pregnancy-promoting recommendations.

You can use these strategies on their own to increase your chances of becoming pregnant. If you are pursuing assisted reproduction, they offer easy ways to boost the chances it will succeed.

We wish we could guarantee that following the Fertility Diet strategies will lead to a pregnancy. But we can't do that any more than a doctor can guarantee you will have a baby following IVF, GIFT, or any other assisted reproduction procedure. And we can safely say that the Fertility Diet strategies won't work for couples who are having trouble getting pregnant because the woman has blocked fallopian tubes or the man's ejaculate is devoid of active sperm cells.

That said, for couples plagued by ovulatory infertility, and possibly other types as well, following our diet, exercise, and weight recommendations increases the odds of conceiving *and* sets the stage for a healthy pregnancy. And over the long term, these changes will benefit your heart, your brain, and the rest of your body.

That's a winning combination, no matter how you look at it.

Update

Science doesn't stand still. It advances knowledge by either adding support for new ideas or gathering evidence to refute them. In the year or so since *The Fertility Diet* was first published, new research has given our work a thumbs-up.

Trans fats, found in many types of stick margarine, fast food, and commercially baked goods, blunt fertility in more ways than just working against ovulation (see Chapter 5). A new report from the Nurses' Health Study shows that women whose diets are high in trans fats are also more likely to develop endometriosis, an overgrowth of the lining of the uterus that can interfere with getting pregnant.[4] A team of Cincinnati researchers showed that trans fats may promote miscarriages by silencing a gene involved in the maturation and function of the placenta.[5] On a positive note, a diet rich in omega-3 fats from fish, walnuts, and other sources appears to help protect against endometriosis.[4]

A recently completed Australian trial supports our recommendations on lifestyle changes. Among women with polycystic ovary syndrome, a condition closely related to ovulatory infertility, changes in diet coupled with an exercise program were more effective than drug therapy for stabilizing menstrual rhythms and reducing its other signs and symptoms, such as excess body hair.[6]

Vitamin D, once thought to be important mainly for bones, is now known to play various roles throughout the body, from the regulation of blood pressure to protection against asthma and several types of cancer. In the Nurses' Health Study, a low level of vitamin D intake was almost, but not quite, a risk factor for ovulatory infertility. A new study from the Albert Einstein College of Medicine suggests that a low intake of vitamin D is associated with ovulatory infertility and that getting plenty of vitamin D (on the order of 1,000 mg a day) may improve ovulatory function.[7]

Not long after *The Fertility Diet* was published, we began hearing from readers and visitors to our website, thefertilitydiet.com. The response has been overwhelmingly positive. Several readers echoed this comment from Stefanie, "Your book has made a huge difference in how I am feeling." Others, such as Sara, appreciated the book because it offered "a lot of really valuable lessons about eating well." The best notes came from readers like Cassie: "I followed your [suggestions] to a 'T' for three months. And then I added my own—I drank a glass of wine a day, relaxed, put it in God's hands, and had intercourse daily or every other day for about a month. Voilà! We are pregnant!"

As we pointed out earlier in this chapter, following the Fertility Diet strategies doesn't guarantee a pregnancy; it won't work miracles; and it isn't for all couples. But it is a simple, inexpensive way to help nature, or modern medicine, take its course.

Chapter 2

Missed Conceptions

Every new life starts with two seemingly simple events. First, an active sperm burrows into a perfectly mature egg. Then the resulting fertilized egg nestles into the specially prepared lining of the uterus and begins to grow.

The key phrase in that description is "seemingly simple." Dozens of steps influenced by a cascade of carefully timed hormones are needed to make and mature eggs and sperm. Their union is both a mad dash and a complex dance, choreographed by hormones, physiology, and environmental cues.

Given the complexity of conception, it's no wonder that infertility has beset couples for as long as they have been trying to have children. In ancient Egypt, infertility was common enough and public enough for the Egyptians to have a popular goddess of infertility, named Nephtys.[1] The biblical story of Sarah's desperate quest for a child, which finally ended with the birth of Isaac when she was ninety, is a tale of infertility, hope, disbelief, and divine intervention. Through the ages, healers and frauds have come up with various remedies for infertility, ranging from poultices of nettles and potions of mare's milk and rabbit blood to electrically charged beds guaranteed to bless their users with progeny.

Today, an estimated six million American couples have trouble conceiving. Age is one factor. Many couples delay having a baby until they are financially ready or have established themselves in their professions. Waiting, though, decreases the odds of conceiving and increases the chances of having a miscarriage, as Figure 2.1 shows. Sexually transmitted diseases such as chlamydia and gonorrhea, which are on the upswing, can cause or contribute to infertility. The linked epidemics of obesity and diabetes sweeping the country have reproductive repercussions. Environmental contaminants known as endocrine disruptors appear to affect fertility in women and men. Stress and anxiety, both in general and about fertility, can also interfere with getting pregnant.

▶Conception Basics

Before delving into infertility and its causes, let's set the stage with a quick review of the main things that need to happen for conception to

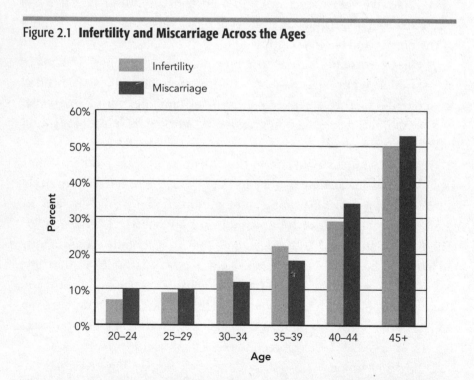

Figure 2.1 **Infertility and Miscarriage Across the Ages**

The longer a couple waits to have a child, the longer they may wait to have a child. Fewer than 10 percent of women in their early twenties have issues with infertility, compared to nearly 30 percent of those in their early forties and half or more of those over age forty-five. Miscarriage also becomes more common with age, compounding the problem of having a baby.

Source: American Society for Reproductive Medicine.

occur. You may remember a lot of this from high school biology class. If not, don't panic—there's no quiz at the end.

All About Eggs

The human egg, or ovum, is one of the largest cells in a woman's body. At a diameter of 150 microns (0.006 inch), it's the size of a pencil point. Girls are born with about two million immature eggs evenly divided between two almond-sized ovaries. (See Figure 2.2.) Between birth and puberty, most of these immature eggs die off, leaving a mere three hundred thousand for the ensuing four hundred reproductive cycles.

Starting at puberty, every twenty-eight days or so, pulses of hormones signal a cluster of eggs in one of the ovaries to mature. In young

Figure 2.2 **Female Reproductive System**

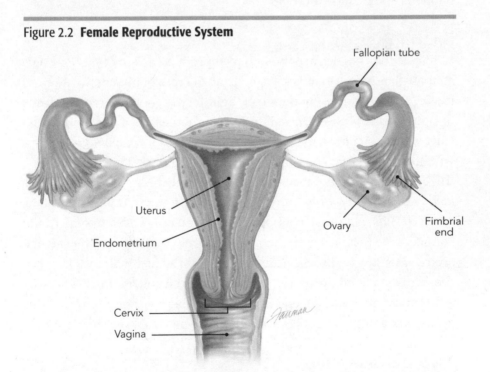

The elongated pyramid of the uterus sits at the center of a woman's reproductive system. Two almond-sized ovaries, one on either side of the uterus, contain thousands of immature eggs. When an egg matures during a menstrual cycle, the ovary releases it into the nearby fallopian tube. The cervix (its name comes from the Latin term for *neck*) is the lower, narrow portion of the uterus where it joins with the top of the vagina.

women, four to ten eggs may begin to develop; in older women, as few as one or two. Each of these activated eggs develops inside its own tiny fluid-filled sac, called a follicle. One egg almost always becomes dominant, while the others fade away and disappear. (Twins or triplets get their start when two or three eggs dominate and mature.) Commanded by a final gust of hormones, the dominant follicle bursts, ejecting its tiny egg toward the beginning of the fallopian tube. This is the moment of ovulation.

Fingerlike fimbria catch the egg and coax it into the fallopian tube. Rhythmically beating cilia ease the ovum along the four-inch tube (the equivalent of a half-mile trek for the average-sized person) toward its opening into the uterus. If fertilization is going to happen, it usually happens in the fallopian tube.

Sperm Factory

In males, the testicles are the hub of reproductive activity. These egg-shaped glands churn out sperm cells at the rate of about one hundred million a day. The sperm-making machinery is contained in hundreds of tightly coiled tubes, the seminiferous tubules. As a new sperm cell travels through one of these tubules, it develops a compact head and a whiplike tail. The juvenile sperm eventually emerges into another tube, the epididymis, where it matures for several weeks. The epididymis also acts as a kind of holding tank. During a man's orgasm, millions of sperm rush out of the epididymis and along the vas deferens, which connects the testicles with the penis. As they hurtle along the vas deferens, they are bathed in a fluid made by the seminal vesicles. The prostate gland and Cowper's gland get into the act, adding lubricating fluids and more nourishment. Strong muscular contractions speed this milky mix along the urethra and out of the penis. (See Figure 2.3.)

Two Become One

During intercourse, a man's ejaculation propels as many as five hundred million madly swimming sperm into the vagina. Guided by chemical signals from the egg—perhaps the most important perfume of sex—they thrash their way into the mucus that protects the cervix and fight their way into the uterus. Some get trapped in the mucus,

Figure 2.3 **Male Reproductive System**

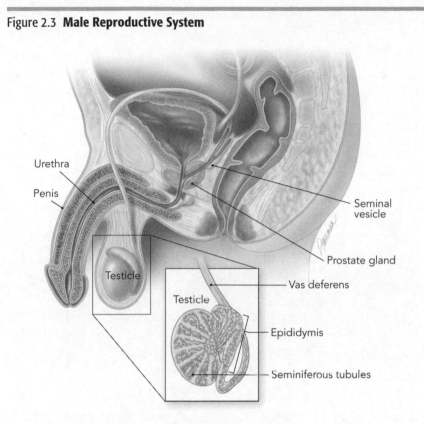

Urethra

Penis

Seminal
vesicle

Testicle

Prostate gland

Testicle

Vas deferens

Epididymis

Seminiferous tubules

A man's testicles are the hub of his reproductive system. Sperm cells are made in the long seminiferous tubules coiled inside each testicle. The epididymis transports sperm from the seminiferous tubules to the foot-long vas deferens, which carries them to the penis. Along the way, the seminal vesicles produce a fluid that, with sperm cells and other fluids from the testicles, creates semen.

some lose their way, some run out of steam. If all the planets are in alignment, a hundred or so sperm manage to navigate their way into the fallopian tubes, only one of which is holding a mature egg. (See Figure 2.4.)

Here's where the dance really begins. The egg, long portrayed as a passive damsel patiently awaiting her knight, plays an active role in their meeting.[2] Attracted by the egg's chemical signals, nearby sperm thrash closer. The egg sends out filaments of protein that guide one or more sperm (or reel them in, depending on your point of view) through the

Figure 2.4 **Steps of Conception**

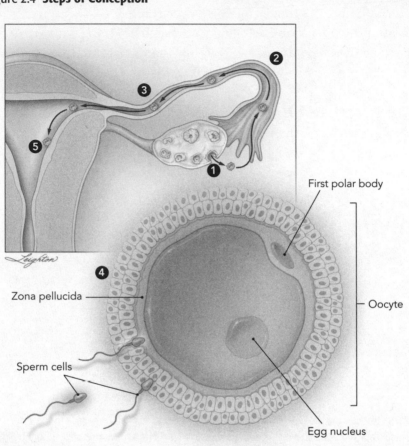

The meeting of egg (oocyte) and sperm is the end of one long journey and, with luck, the beginning of another. (1) It starts with an ovary's release of a mature egg that is gathered in by the fimbrial end of the fallopian tube. (2) The egg floats through the fallopian tube toward the uterus. (3) Somewhere along the way, it meets one or more sperm cells that have traveled from the vagina through the cervix and uterus, attracted by the true perfume of sex—subtle chemical signals given off by the egg. (4) The culmination of the complex dance between egg and sperm occurs when one sperm burrows into the egg and delivers its cargo of twenty-three chromosomes into the egg's nucleus. They match up one for one with the egg's twenty-three chromosomes. (5) The fertilized egg floats out of the fallopian tube and into the uterus, where it nestles into the specially prepared endometrium.

jellylike cumulus surrounding the egg. Held firmly in place, the sperm latch onto the egg's tough *zona pellucida* (Latin for "glassy layer") and release proteins capable of chewing through it. The first sperm to get inside delivers its cargo—twenty-three spindly chromosomes, which match up one for one with the egg's twenty-three chromosomes.

The Fertilized Egg's Journey

After a few hours, the transformed egg starts its slow voyage out of the fallopian tube and into the uterus. It grows and divides as it floats along. Within five days, it's a ball of about two hundred cells. This ball, called a blastocyst, secretes enzymes that erode the top layer of the endometrium (the lining of the uterus), which has become swollen with new blood vessels in preparation for just such an occupant. The blastocyst then settles into the endometrium and begins making connections with these new blood vessels. Thus begins the physical link between mother and child that, if all goes well, ends with birth nine months later.

The Complex Role of Hormones

If egg and sperm are the primary dancers in this ballet, hormones make the music that guides their rhythm and movements. A small part of the brain called the hypothalamus conducts the fertilization dance.

Hormones are chemical messengers made in one part of the body that act on tissues or cells somewhere else. The hormone insulin, for example, is made in the pancreas but acts throughout the body, mainly on muscle cells, telling them to grab sugar from the bloodstream. The key reproductive hormones are gonadotropin-releasing hormone (GnRH), follicle-stimulating hormone (FSH), luteinizing hormone (LH), estrogen, progesterone, and testosterone. (See Figure 2.5 for the main reproductive hormones in women.)

The hypothalamus is an almond-sized section of the brain that sits directly behind the eyes. One of its many jobs is to send out pulses of GnRH. This hormone tells the pituitary gland, which hangs by a stalk from the hypothalamus, to release two other hormones—FSH and LH—into the bloodstream. These two oversee the cycle of reproduction in women and men.

Figure 2.5 **Key Reproductive Hormones in Women**

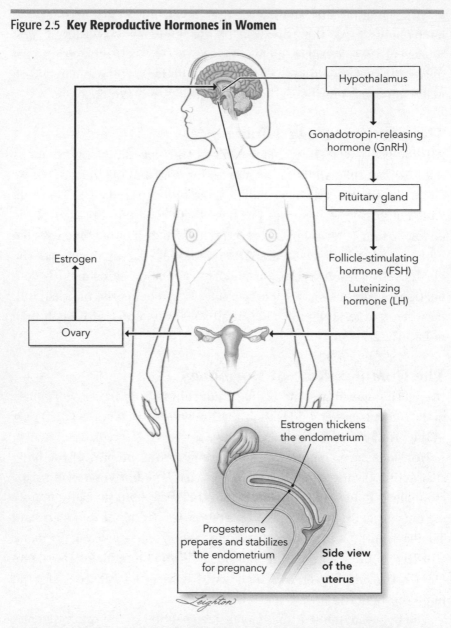

Numerous hormones and cell-signaling molecules are involved in the monthly cycle of ovulation and preparation for a possible pregnancy. The five main hormones are gonadotropin-releasing hormone (GnRH), follicle-stimulating hormone (FSH), luteinizing hormone (LH), estrogen, and progesterone. GnRH is made in the hypothalamus. It stimulates the pituitary gland to make FSH and LH. These two work together to mature and release an egg. One of the many functions of estrogen and progesterone is to prepare the endometrium (the lining of the uterus) for a possible pregnancy.

In women, FSH provokes a cluster of eggs to begin maturing. LH works with FSH to ripen an egg. One way it does this is by stimulating theca cells in the ovary to make androgens (male sex hormones) and other substances that are the precursors for estradiol, the main form of estrogen. A surge in production of LH triggers ovulation. Afterward, this hormone is responsible for converting the eggless follicle into the *corpus luteum* (Latin for "yellow body"), which is necessary for preparing the endometrium for a possible pregnancy.

Estrogen plays many different roles in reproduction. Follicles secrete it as they mature. The pituitary gland responds to the rise in estrogen by cutting back on its production of FSH, an action that slows and then stops the growth of all but the most advanced follicle. At the same time, it stimulates the endometrium to thicken. Estrogen is also essential for maintaining the reproductive organs and female sex characteristics.

Progesterone comes mainly from the corpus luteum. Under instructions from LH, the corpus luteum generates progesterone, which helps prepare the endometrium for a fertilized egg by stimulating the growth of new blood vessels.

A woman's body produces varying amounts of these hormones throughout her menstrual cycle. They generally peak just before ovulation and then fall off and slowly rise again. (See Figure 2.6.)

In men, FSH keeps the sperm-making machinery up and running, while LH prompts the testicles to make testosterone, the main male sex hormone. Testosterone helps stimulate the formation of new sperm cells, maintains the function of the reproductive organs, and keeps the sex drive alive.

Although FSH and LH do completely different things in women and men, they are named after their actions in women, because they were first discovered in women.

A host of other hormones or their chaperones play roles in the maturation of eggs and sperm, the preparation for ovulation and ejaculation, the union of sperm and egg, and the development of the fertilized egg. Several of these are important for understanding how diet can affect fertility.

Figure 2.6 **Changes Across the Menstrual Cycle**

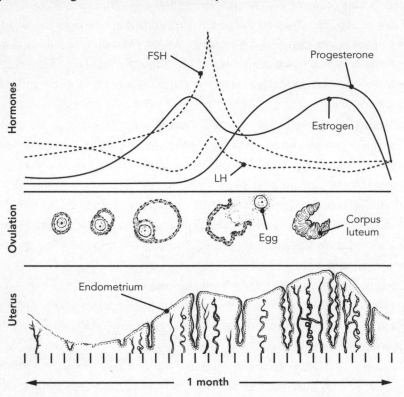

A lot happens during a menstrual cycle. At the beginning (day 1 is considered to be the first day of menstrual bleeding), hormone levels are generally low. FSH gradually rises, while LH drifts downward. These changes spur one follicle to mature and the endometrium (the lining of the uterus) to begin to thicken in preparation for a possible pregnancy. A surge in FSH and LH triggers ovulation. Production of estrogen and progesterone stimulate further growth and development of the endometrium. If the egg is not fertilized, levels of estrogen and progesterone plummet, causing the body to shed the blood-vessel-rich endometrium.

■ **Sex hormone binding globulin.** Sex hormones generally don't float freely through the bloodstream but are escorted by a protein known as sex hormone binding globulin. This chaperone makes sure sex hormones don't exert their biological effects all the time and on all tissues. Sex hormone binding globulin latches onto testosterone more strongly than it does to estrogen. Levels of this protein in circulation change in response to other hormones, as well as to diet, lifestyle, and disease. An increase in estrogen or thyroid hormone increases the body's production of sex hormone binding globulin, which, in turn, decreases the amount of free testosterone. Increases in testosterone or other androgens, insulin, growth hormone, and insulin-like growth factor-1 decrease the amount of sex hormone binding globulin, and this increases free testosterone.

■ **Insulin.** Every cell in the body uses sugar—particularly the sugar glucose—as a source of energy. Yet glucose can't flow freely into cells. Instead, it must pass through a molecular gate that only insulin can open. This hormone is made by cells in the pancreas when blood sugar levels rise above a certain carefully controlled level. If these cells falter in their ability to produce insulin, or if muscle cells become resistant to its effect, sugar builds up in the bloodstream. That's the hallmark of type 2 diabetes, an increasingly common disease in the United States and around the world. More insulin in the bloodstream depresses the production of sex hormone binding globulin. This leads to higher amounts of circulating free testosterone, which can have unwanted effects on fertility and physiology.

■ **Insulin-like growth factor-1.** This growth hormone tells cells to grow and divide. Insulin-like growth factor-1 affects almost every kind of cell in the body, especially those in muscle, cartilage, bone, liver, kidney, nerves, skin, and lungs. It is chemically similar to insulin (hence the name) and sometimes even acts like it. Like insulin, it can affect reproduction by decreasing the amount of circulating sex hormone binding globulin, which increases the amount of free testosterone.

■ **Leptin.** A gene known as *ob* (for obesity) makes a hormone called leptin. The name is derived from the Greek word *leptos*, meaning "thin." The body's fat cells make leptin and dump it into the bloodstream when they begin to swell with fat after a meal or snack. The hormone's message is basically, "You have eaten enough; now start burning what you've eaten." A low level of leptin conveys the opposite message. It tells the body to conserve energy, and it triggers hunger.

Because leptin probably evolved as a way of keeping tabs on fat stores, it is involved in regulating many systems throughout the body, including the reproductive system. In mice, a starvation-induced fall in leptin lowers the body temperature to conserve energy, increases production of stress hormones, and turns down reproduction by dampening ovulation in females and sperm production and mating behavior in males. These changes may improve the chances of surviving without food. Similar changes may occur in very active women who lose a lot of their body fat—ovulation starts to fail and eventually stops altogether. In the opposite direction, young girls need to accumulate enough fat tissue before puberty can begin. It is possible that the amount of leptin reaching the brain from fat cells influences both of these responses.

■ **Adiponectin.** Body fat used to be thought of as little more than inert storage tissue. It's turning out to be anything but. Fat cells, more formally known as adipocytes, churn out a variety of hormones and cell-signaling molecules known as cytokines. Adiponectin is secreted exclusively by fat cells and is the most abundant protein they make. It helps turn on chemical pathways that burn fats. It also helps make cells more sensitive to insulin, which may enhance ovulation. Adiponectin may also have anti-inflammatory effects on cells lining the walls of blood vessels. Curiously, the more weight you gain, the less adiponectin your fat cells make. This drop-off may be one reason why people who are overweight tend to be resistant to insulin.

▶What Can Go Wrong

Conception requires the careful coordination of many key events, actions, and hormones. It may not be quite as complicated as launching the space shuttle, but it comes pretty close.

A delay or problem in a single step, like ovulation in a woman or sperm motility in a man, can block conception or make it even less likely to happen than it already is. So can too much of one hormone or too little of another. The American Society for Reproductive Medicine estimates that one-third of all cases of infertility can be chalked up to male factors and another third to female factors. In the remaining third, either both partners have problems that limit fertility or the problem is labeled as "unexplained" since no obvious fertility-hindering condition can be found in either partner. There are so many ways to derail conception that finding the problem, and correcting it, can be tricky.

Female Factors

Barriers to pregnancy in women range from physical problems such as blocked fallopian tubes to hormonal imbalances.

■ **Ovulation disorders.** LH, FSH, and estrogen are needed for the maturation and release of an egg from the ovary (ovulation). Poorly timed release of these hormones, or inappropriate amounts of them, can interfere with ovulation. Other hormones can also throw it off. Ovulatory problems are a common cause of infertility in women and contribute to one-quarter or more of all cases of infertility.

■ **Polycystic ovaries.** As many as one in ten women have a condition known as polycystic ovary syndrome (PCOS). This health problem can affect a woman's menstrual cycle and fertility and is the most common cause of ovulatory infertility. Because PCOS is such an important contributor to ovulatory infertility, we describe it more fully later in this chapter, along with important advances that are improving the chances of successful pregnancies in women with it.

■ **Disorders of the uterus and cervix.** Fibroids, polyps, and other growths on the wall of the uterus can prevent a fertilized egg from nestling into and then attaching to the uterine wall. An abnormally shaped cervix or cervical mucus that is too thick or hostile to sperm can form physical barriers that keep sperm from a date with an egg in the privacy of a fallopian tube.

■ **Damage to the fallopian tube.** A full or partial blockage of the fallopian tube can interfere with conception by preventing sperm from entering. A common cause of this kind of obstruction is pelvic inflammatory disease, which is a complication of chlamydia, gonorrhea, or other sexually transmitted diseases. Blocked tubes can also result from scarring or adhesions from surgery, as well as inflammation from other viral or bacterial infections.

■ **Endometriosis.** The endometrium is a layer of tissue that lines the inside of the uterus. In some women, endometrial tissue grows where it isn't supposed to—in the ovaries, on the outside surface of the uterus, around the fallopian tubes, and in the spaces between the bladder, uterus, and rectum. This misplaced tissue tends to behave like normal endometrial tissue, thickening and shrinking in response to the monthly cycle of female hormones. This can be very painful. By covering or growing into the ovaries, or by distorting or blocking the fallopian tubes, endometriosis can also hinder conception or the development of a fertilized egg.

■ **Immune attack.** The immune system is ever vigilant for foreign invaders. Luckily for our species, the immune systems of most women don't attack sperm the same way they attack viruses or bacteria, or at least they don't mount permanent campaigns against them. In some women, though, antisperm antibodies in the cervical mucus overwhelm sperm, slowing them down or disabling them until they are destroyed by white blood cells. In other women, the immune system attacks the fertilized egg or embryo.

Polycystic Ovary Syndrome. In 1935, two Chicago gynecologists wrote about an "unusual" cluster of symptoms in seven of their patients: irregular or nonexistent menstrual periods, excess facial and body hair, and enlarged ovaries filled with small cysts. Little did these doctors, Irving Stein and Michael Leventhal, know that what they were describing was a hormonal hurricane that is one of the most common causes of infertility. It is also an early indicator of heightened risk for type 2 diabetes, heart disease, and possibly some types of cancer.

The condition, initially called Stein-Leventhal syndrome, is now known as polycystic ovary syndrome (PCOS). (See Figure 2.7.) It has also been called syndrome O and syndrome XX. No one really knows how common PCOS is. In the United States, it affects somewhere between 5 percent and 10 percent of women. A new study from Spain puts the figure at more than 25 percent for women who are seriously overweight.

PCOS isn't exactly a disease. It's a syndrome—a collection of signs and symptoms stemming from other underlying problems or diseases. A woman has PCOS if she has two of the following:

- High levels of androgens (male hormones) detected by a blood test or by features such as too much body or facial hair, thinning hair on the scalp, or acne
- Problems with ovulation, which usually appear as long or irregular menstrual cycles, cycles without ovulation, or no periods at all
- Enlarged ovaries that have many small cysts

Figure 2.7 **A Polycystic Ovary**

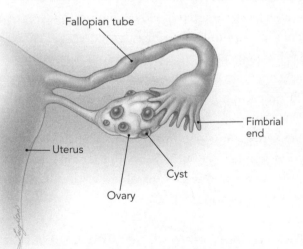

In women with polycystic ovary syndrome (PCOS), maturing follicles can remain trapped in the ovary instead of being released at ovulation. These unreleased follicles create multiple small cysts (polycystic, in doctorspeak) throughout the ovary.

Other features that aren't considered to be proof positive of PCOS, but that commonly occur in women with the condition, include above-normal levels of LH; excess weight, especially around the midsection; and resistance to the actions of insulin.

In some women, the signs and symptoms are relatively easy to detect. They can also be so subtle, or invisible, that many women aren't aware they have PCOS.

These outward signs are wrought by a hormone storm that affects fertility and long-term health. The most devastating are resistance to insulin and the overproduction of male sex hormones. They are largely responsible for the cosmetic, reproductive, and long-term health effects associated with PCOS.

Problems with Insulin. A hallmark of PCOS is an insensitivity to the life-sustaining signals of insulin. This hormone, which is secreted by the pancreas, helps cells absorb blood sugar (glucose) from the bloodstream, something they can't do on their own. Insulin resistance occurs when cells need more and more insulin to do the job. As a result, levels of both blood sugar and insulin climb higher than they should. Like a spark that starts a slow, smoldering fire, resistance to insulin touches off a bundle of unhealthy metabolic changes. In women with PCOS—and probably in many without it—too much insulin leads to a derangement of sex hormones that can stop ovulation in its tracks.

Chronically high levels of insulin and insulin-like growth factor-1 (IGF-1) stimulate cells in the ovary to overproduce male hormones. At the same time, insulin and IGF-1 block the liver from making sex hormone binding globulin. As its amount in circulation dwindles, more and more free androgens capable of stimulating a variety of tissues appear in the bloodstream.

Testosterone Overload. In the ovaries, cells known as theca cells convert cholesterol into testosterone and other androgens. Some of these are converted into estradiol. Small amounts of androgens also promote the monthly growth and early maturation of follicles. In women with PCOS, high levels of insulin and insulin-like growth factor-1 put the androgen-making process into overdrive, turning a trickle of testosterone into a flood. Too much yang and not enough yin hurries follicles to the brink of maturation and then abruptly shuts down their development. The end result? No egg is released.

In addition to preventing ovulation, the extra androgens made by the theca cells get into the bloodstream. As they circulate through the body, they stimulate the growth of body hair, thin the hair on the scalp, and trigger acne.

Three Paths to Fertility and Good Health. PCOS was initially thought of as a fertility problem. We now know that the hormonal imbalances that cause or accompany it pose equally serious risks to long-term health. Fortunately, the strategies that improve ovulation in women with PCOS are the same ones that reduce facial and body hair and prevent heart disease, type 2 diabetes, and other long-term consequences. The three key steps are weight loss, diet, and insulin-sensitizing medications.

■ **Weight loss.** A number of studies have shown that women with PCOS who are overweight can do wonders for themselves by losing weight. A loss of around 5 percent of one's starting weight can make a big difference.[3] For someone weighing 160 pounds, that's eight pounds. (More, of course, is even better.) This modest amount of weight loss improves the body's sensitivity to insulin, lowers levels of male hormones, improves menstrual regularity and ovulation, and helps clear up acne and reduce excess facial and body hair. Losing weight isn't easy for most people, but it may be even more difficult for women with PCOS. That's because high levels of androgens can increase appetite, and insulin resistance may hinder weight loss.

There hasn't been much research on the best weight-loss strategies for women with PCOS. Cutting calories is a must, though how to do this is a matter of personal preference, as we describe in Chapter 10. Exercise is essential.

■ **Diet.** There isn't much definitive knowledge yet about the effects of different foods and diet strategies in women with PCOS. Two small studies comparing high-protein weight-loss diets to standard ones showed that *any* weight loss improved measures of reproductive function. How the volunteers got there didn't much matter. Another study showed no differences in menstrual cycle regularity between women asked to follow a high-protein diet and those asked to follow a low-protein diet. A fourth showed that increasing the intake of polyunsaturated fat by eating four ounces of walnuts a day and decreasing saturated fat had no effect on levels of insulin, testosterone, LH, or FSH. And although the diet did improve one blood marker for ovulation, only two of the seventeen volunteers had menstrual patterns that suggested ovulation.

Choosing whole, intact grains that are high in fiber and other slowly digested carbohydrates while minimizing rapidly digested carbs and sugared sodas is a sensible strategy.[4] It will help keep blood sugar and insulin under control, which may reduce food cravings. Vegetables, fruits, beans, and nuts are also excellent ways to keep blood sugar in check.

■ **Medications.** Two classes of drugs traditionally used to treat diabetes have been used to improve blood sugar and promote ovulation in women with PCOS. Metformin (generic and Glucophage) cuts down on the liver's release of stored glucose. This means the pancreas doesn't need to make as much insulin. With less insulin in circulation, the ovaries generate less testosterone and other androgens, which is good for ovulation. Diabetes drugs known as thiazolidinediones help muscle, liver, and fat cells respond more efficiently to insulin. This helps keep blood sugar levels in check after a meal or snack. The two thiazolidinediones in use today are rosiglitazone (Avandia) and pioglitazone (Actos). In small trials, metformin, rosiglitazone, and pioglitazone have lowered insulin and androgen levels and improved ovulation in women with PCOS.

None of the Fertility Diet recommendations that improve sensitivity to insulin—switching from rapidly digested carbohydrates to whole grains and other slowly digested carbohydrates, cutting out trans fats and consuming more unsaturated fats, and eating more plant protein and less animal protein—have been rigorously tested in women with PCOS. When they are, we bet they will work, because each of these can aid in weight loss and improve sensitivity to insulin. What's more, a diet and exercise approach will probably turn out to be more effective than medications, just as it is more effective than drug therapy at preventing diabetes.

Male Factors

The quantity and quality of sperm are the main reproductive issues in men. Making too few sperm or sperm that are listless, physically handicapped, or poor swimmers can stem from physical problems, such as blocked spermatic cords or infection, to lifestyle factors, such as smoking or abuse of steroids or other drugs.

■ **Low sperm count.** Although it takes only one sperm to fertilize an egg, the odds of any single sperm reaching an egg are mighty low. The more sperm released into the vagina during intercourse, the greater the odds that one will have enough stamina, elude the traps, head in the right direction, and hook up with an egg. A low sperm count is defined as fewer than twenty million sperm per milliliter of semen. This isn't an absolute, though, since men with lower counts have fathered children, while men with higher counts can be infertile.

■ **Sperm defects.** Abnormalities in the shape of sperm or their ability to swim can delay or prevent conception. These can be due to hormonal imbalances, infection, or a variety of other causes.

■ **Twisted tubes.** In some men, one or both spermatic cords are so twisted that sperm have trouble making their way from the testicles to the penis. Injuries and some sexually transmitted diseases can cause this problem. Another physical impediment to fertility is a varicocele—a dilation in veins that drain blood from the testicles. Because varicoceles are sometimes associated with sperm abnormalities, they are often surgically repaired in men with fertility problems. Whether fixing varicoceles actually improves fertility, though, is controversial.

■ **Immune attack.** Some men make antibodies against their own sperm. This civil war makes sperm unfit for fertilization.

Couple Factors

About one-third of the time, infertility arises from a problem in both partners or when both check out fine on all the standard tests and even some very high-tech ones. In some cases, unexplained infertility stems from an undiagnosed condition, such as celiac disease (see Chapter 8). In others, it remains a true mystery.

One relatively simple couple factor is mistimed intercourse. For most women, there's a seven-day window of opportunity for conception. It generally opens six days before ovulation starts, peaks on the day of ovulation, and closes the day after.[5] During this time frame, the chances of conception get better and better the closer to ovulation you have intercourse. Knowing when the window opens isn't always easy. Some women can make a good guess based on their cycle length and regularity. Others rely on a change in cervical mucus, a tiny spike in body temperature (using a basal body temperature thermometer), or ovulation predictor kits that detect the surge in LH just before ovulation to know when their most fertile days are.

▶When Does "Trying" Segue into Infertility?

How long does it usually take to get pregnant? Several large studies that have followed couples from the time they stop using contraceptives show that about one-third become pregnant in the first month. By three months, half are pregnant. That rises to 80 percent by six months and 90 percent by the end of a year. These numbers are the basis for the common definition of infertility: the inability to conceive after one full year of regular intercourse without the use of contraception. But because the majority of pregnancies occur within the first six months of trying, some doctors recommend that couples undergo a workup for infertility after six months of trying, especially when the woman is age thirty-five or older.

Does not getting pregnant within a year mean you won't manage to do it without treatment? No. Some couples who try for much longer than a year without seeking medical help eventually get pregnant. There aren't good numbers on this. One older study showed that about one-third of couples who didn't get pregnant within a year of trying eventually did over a three-year period.

Secondary Infertility

When most people hear "infertility," they think immediately of childless couples yearning for a baby. Yet infertility also affects a surprising number of couples who already have a child, or more than one, and want more. This can be just as unsettling and emotionally draining as primary infertility.

Although secondary infertility is quite common, it tends to be an invisible, or at least less acknowledged, problem. Couples are less likely to seek advice or help for secondary infertility, especially when their first child was conceived quickly. But past fertility doesn't guarantee future children. In general, secondary infertility stems from the same causes as primary infertility and responds to the same fertility-boosting strategies.

Removing the "In" from Infertile

If you have been trying to have a baby for at least a year and the standard approach—having sex often—isn't working, don't hesitate to see a doctor. Go even sooner if you are over age thirty-five. That's the advice from the American Society for Reproductive Medicine, the American College of Obstetricians and Gynecologists, and other medical organizations.

A visit with a reproductive specialist may pinpoint what's getting in your way. It could be something that requires medical attention, like diabetes, celiac disease, an underactive thyroid gland, or excess weight. Or it could be something that's correctable with a minor surgical procedure, like opening a blocked fallopian tube, removing endometriosis or fibroids, or fixing varicose veins in the scrotum. It is also possible the doctor might recommend a high-tech procedure such as in vitro fertilization (IVF), intracytoplasmic sperm injection (ICSI), or gamete intrafallopian tube transfer (GIFT).

Those are time-tested technologies that have worked for more than a million couples. But don't overlook lower-tech, do-it-yourself approaches first. If you smoke, quitting may help speed a pregnancy.

Smokers—both women and men—are more likely than nonsmokers to be infertile, and it takes them longer to conceive.[6] Meditation or other stress-busting practices can also improve fertility.[7]

The diet and exercise strategies we describe in Chapters 4 through 11 offer a powerful do-it-yourself plan for boosting your fertility. The steps we recommend can be used on their own or as a booster for assisted reproduction technologies. Keep in mind, though, that diet, exercise, smoking cessation, stress reduction, and other self-help approaches can't beat a blocked fallopian tube or the condition known as azoospermia (few or no active sperm in semen).

Chapter 3

A Diet for All Ages

Healthy eating used to be so simple: if you ate, you were healthy; if you didn't, you weren't. Of course, those were the days when the average adult was lucky to celebrate a fortieth birthday. Now that we can reasonably expect to live to eighty or beyond, healthy eating is no longer quite so straightforward. It isn't enough just to get the calories you need to power your body, build it, and repair it, because the foods that supply these calories govern the health of your heart, influence whether or not you will develop cancer, or determine if you will end up with osteoporosis, age-related eye or memory loss, or a host of other chronic conditions.

But which foods, or nutrients, are best?

For years, guidelines for healthy eating have been ruled by the stick (what you *shouldn't* eat) rather than the carrot (what you *should* eat). Diets were more about deprivation than delight. This kind of approach can spoil anyone's appetite and break up what should be an enjoyable relationship with food.

Now there is a new approach *based on sound science* that stresses adding more of what's good for you rather than telling you what to avoid. As you will see, it doesn't focus on a single miracle food or dietary demon. Instead, it offers a mixture with an abundance of healthy choices. This approach is captured in the Healthy Eating Pyramid, shown in Figure 3.1. It is built from these key building blocks:

Figure 3.1 **Healthy Eating Pyramid for Fertility**

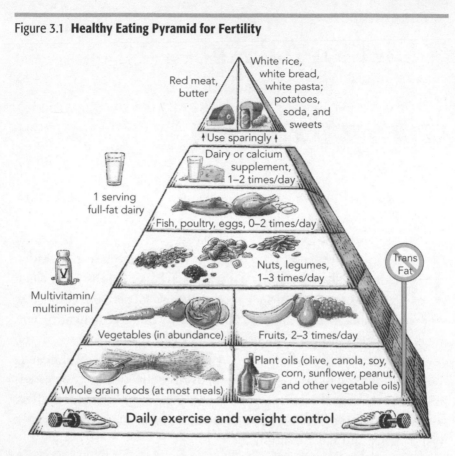

The Healthy Eating Pyramid is based on the best scientific advice available today. It encourages you to make whole grains, healthful unsaturated fats, whole fruits, and vegetables the foundation of your diet, supplemented by beans, nuts, fish, poultry, and eggs. Red meat and rapidly digested carbohydrates occupy the "use sparingly" pyramid penthouse. Adapting this strategy for fertility means including a daily serving or two of whole milk or full-fat dairy and taking a prenatal supplement that contains 400 mcg of folic acid and 40 to 80 mg of iron.

Source: Adapted from *Eat, Drink, and Be Healthy* by Walter C. Willett with Patrick J. Skerrett, Free Press, 2005.

more fruits and vegetables, good fats, good sources of carbohydrates, healthy protein, and smart beverage choices. The advice embodied in the Healthy Eating Pyramid works for Generation Xers, baby boomers, and the oldest old. Using it as a guide can help you lengthen your life and start a new one.

Information Overload

In 1951, the venerable *Joy of Cooking* summed up the then-current thinking on healthy eating this way:

> Two fruits and three vegetables daily. Good protein from meat, dairy products, eggs, fish, dried peas, and beans. Baked goods made with whole grains and flavored with brown sugar or molasses.

Given the limited information available at the time on human nutrition, *Joy*'s advice was pretty good.

Back then, nutrition was a sluggish backwater of medical research. Today it is a fast-flowing river, flooding an interested public with new findings almost daily. This explosion in research is wonderful because the findings nudge us closer to a more complete understanding of how food and diet influence health and disease. But there's a downside that stems from the jerky nature of science. Studies contradict each other, animal studies may not apply to humans, and what is learned today may change in the light of tomorrow's advances in chemistry or genetics. We hear about these baby steps in the news. All too often they are presented as breakthroughs or flip-flops, rather than the inevitable give-and-take of the scientific method.

Thumb through the magazines at your grocery store the next time you are waiting to check out and you'll get an idea of the disorder of science and scientific communication. You might learn that soy is your key to good health—or to getting breast cancer. That you should eat more fish—or stay away from it because it might contain mercury. That carbohydrates are good for you—or the cause of those extra pounds you are carrying. A chemical found in cranberries stops cancer, but eating fruits and vegetables doesn't fight cancer.

All this "news" creates the illusion of confusion. That's a shame because there are now enough solid strands of evidence from reliable sources to weave simple but compelling recommendations about diet.

The Dietary Guidelines for Americans,[1] a document updated every five years by the U.S. Department of Agriculture, offers a fairly good summary of this evidence. It isn't entirely objective, though, coming from the arm of the federal government charged with promoting American agriculture rather than public health. That's why two of us (Dr. Willett with Skerrett) wrote *Eat, Drink, and Be Healthy: The Harvard Medical School Guide to Healthy Eating*.[2] It offers a look at the "new nutrition" that is beholden to none. In this chapter, we summarize this eating strategy. Chapters 4 through 11 focus on specific fertility-boosting food types or nutrients that perfectly complement the Healthy Eating Pyramid.

Some of the recommendations may surprise you, some may echo what your mother told you as a kid, and some you will recognize as plain common sense. But all of them are based on the strongest, most consistent evidence available today.

▶Carb Loading

Carbohydrates were once the Rodney Dangerfields of nutrients—they didn't get much respect. Everyone knew they provided fuel, some building blocks, and maybe some fiber. And they formed the safe base of the USDA's poorly built Food Pyramid. But many nutrition experts didn't think they exerted a powerful influence on health. That's certainly changed. The Atkins, South Beach, and other "no-carb" diets put carbohydrates on the hot seat, blaming carbs as the villain for weight gain and poor health. Millions of Americans turned their backs on bread, pasta, and even some fruits and vegetables. Even as that fad has ebbed away, solid research from around the globe has shown that, as is the case for fat, there are good carbs and bad carbs. Choosing the right kinds can help set the course for your long-term health.

What are the right kinds? Those in whole fruits, vegetables, whole grains, and beans. Eating these excellent sources of carbohydrates and cutting back on highly refined and highly processed grains can reduce your chances of having a heart attack or stroke, dying of cardiovascular disease, or developing type 2 diabetes, some forms of cancer, and other chronic conditions.

Focusing on these good carbs has a fertility payoff as well. In the Nurses' Health Study, women who had never had a child and whose diets were poor in whole grains and other sources of good carbohydrate were 55 percent more likely to have had trouble with ovulatory infertility than women whose diets included grains that were mostly whole.

Good Carbs, Bad Carbs

What makes one food a better source of carbohydrate than another? One important yardstick is how they affect blood sugar. The body turns bad carbs into blood sugar in a flash. The pancreas responds by churning out a lot of insulin, which can drive down blood sugar so fast and so far that your body starts sending out hunger signals. If you reach for more easily digested carbohydrates, the cycle starts all over again. This blood sugar roller coaster can cause cells to become resistant to insulin's "open up for sugar" signal, forcing the pancreas to constantly make extra insulin. Over the long term, this can wear out the pancreas, leading to type 2 diabetes, and result in weight gain.

Oatmeal, beans, vegetables, and other sources of good carbs give up their sugars more reluctantly, making for slower, gentler rises in blood sugar and insulin with lower peaks. This allows you to go longer between meals without feeling hungry.

And what about fertility? The amount of insulin in circulation influences the amount of sex hormone binding globulin, the protein that cloaks testosterone and estrogen in the bloodstream. Because sex hormone binding globulin has a predilection for testosterone over estrogen, less of it in circulation translates into more free—and thus active—testosterone. Too much active testosterone can hinder or even halt ovulation.

Fruits and Vegetables

We won't waste many words telling you something you already know: eating more fruits and vegetables is one of the smartest dietary changes you can make for your health. A diet rich in fruits and vegetables can lower your blood pressure, diminish your chances of having a heart attack or stroke, guard against some cancers, control your weight, delay or prevent age-related memory or vision loss, and keep you regular. That's an impressive list for some of the most delectable and inexpensive foods you can buy (or grow).

When it comes to fruits and vegetables, the two key principles to keep in mind are (1) more and (2) more variety.

You probably know about the 5-a-Day campaign, which encourages us to get a total of five servings of fruits and vegetables a day. We say *aim higher*. Consider five servings a day as a starting point and shoot for more.

It is also a good idea to follow the rainbow, from red tomatoes through orange carrots, yellow squash, green spinach, blueberries, indigo plums, and violet eggplant. The pot of gold at the end of this rainbow is great taste, a host of beneficial nutrients, colorful meals, and better health—something no leprechaun can steal.

Some people don't eat enough fruits and vegetables because they think preparing them is too much work. Others don't know what to do with kale, mango, delicata squash, or kiwifruit and instead rely on the same tired dozen fruits and veggies week after week. If you recognize yourself here, the recipes in Chapter 13 can show you how to cut the work, broaden your vegetal horizons, and create mouth-watering dishes that will have you and anyone you cook for coming back for more. Cookbooks such as *Vegetable Heaven* by Mollie Katzen and Deborah Madison's *Vegetarian Cooking for Everyone* contain recipes that even confirmed carnivores will eat.

▶Debunking Fat Myths

You'd never know it from the all-out assault on dietary fat over the years, but your body needs fat and (gasp) cholesterol, too. Fat provides energy and padding. Cholesterol gives your body the raw materials it needs for cell membranes, the skin surrounding each cell that controls what gets in and what gets out. It is also used to build the sheath that surrounds and protects nerves, vitamin D, sex hormones, and families of important cell-signaling molecules.

Too much of the wrong kind of fat and too much cholesterol in the diet, though, can cause problems. The biggest worry is atherosclerosis, the narrowing and stiffening of blood vessels throughout the body. This plumbing problem, which afflicts most Americans, occurs when LDL (bad) cholesterol accumulates in patches along the inside of artery walls. These fat-laden patches, known as atherosclerotic plaque, can bulge into the channel available for blood flow. This reduces the flow of oxygen-rich blood to the heart muscle, brain, kidneys, legs, or elsewhere. If a plaque bursts open and spews its contents into the bloodstream, the clot that forms to seal the break can cause a heart attack or stroke.

Food contains four main types of fat: monounsaturated, polyunsaturated, saturated, and trans. Since the 1980s, the main message on diet has been the stark and simple "Fat is bad." There wasn't much support for that advice when it was first promoted some twenty-five years ago, and there is even less now.

We have a different message: "fat isn't a four-letter word." The right types can enliven your meals and keep you healthy.

The Good, the Bad, and the In-Between

Given our long brainwashing on fats, many people find it hard to grasp the truth about them: some fats are good for you, and some aren't. Monounsaturated and polyunsaturated fats are utterly good for you. Saturated fats *in moderation* are OK; too much of them aren't good for long-term health, though. Trans fats pose a special hazard to long-term health and fertility.

Mono- and Polyunsaturated Fats. These fats, all liquids at room temperature, have a host of healthful effects in the body. Eating them instead of saturated fats or rapidly digested carbohydrates like white rice, white bread, and potatoes is good for the heart and arteries. They lower LDL (bad) cholesterol without also lowering HDL (good) cholesterol; keep blood from clotting too readily inside arteries, thus guarding against heart attack and stroke; and prevent the heart from sliding into erratic heartbeats, the main cause of sudden death. Unsaturated fats are also important for healthy reproduction. By helping the body control blood sugar and calm inflammation, they can improve your chances of getting pregnant.

One type of polyunsaturated fat worth highlighting is the omega-3 fat family. Omega-3 fats are most abundant in fatty fish, walnuts, and flaxseeds. The human body can't make these fats from scratch, so you have to get them from food. In addition to providing critical building blocks for cells and hormones, they help prevent heart disease and stroke and may protect against some cancers and other chronic conditions. They are also important for the development of a baby's brain before and after birth.

Good sources of monosaturated fats include olive, canola, and other liquid vegetable oils; nuts and seeds; avocados; and fatty, cold-water fish such as salmon or herring.

Saturated Fats. These aren't health builders like their unsaturated cousins. Instead, they are closely connected with how much harmful LDL is in your bloodstream and lodges in your arteries. Limiting your intake of saturated fat is good: going easy on—or avoiding, if you want—red meat and animal fat and vegetable oils like palm and coconut oil. Whole milk and full-fat dairy products are prime sources of saturated fat. Normally they would be on the "have occasionally" list. But if you are trying to get pregnant, a daily serving or two of whole milk or other full-fat dairy foods or a small bowl of ice cream per day works against ovulatory infertility, as we describe in Chapter 7.

Eliminating saturated fats from your diet isn't possible or even worth it. Having them in the right proportion with unsaturated fat is perfectly fine. It's all about balance. Try to keep your saturated fat intake below 8 percent of calories, or less than seventeen grams a day. That's the amount in seven pats of butter, three glasses of regular milk, three slices of cooked bacon, or one Burger King Whopper with Cheese.

Trans Fats. This type of unsaturated fat is great for the food industry and terrible for your arteries. Most of the trans fat in our food comes from chemical plants rather than green plants. It is a by-product of converting liquid vegetable oil into a solid or semisolid by heating it and bubbling hydrogen through it. This process, called partial hydrogenation, yields a fat that doesn't spoil or turn rancid as readily as nonhydrogenated oil. In restaurant deep fryers, it can be used over and over again without breaking down. This stability, along with its low cost, is why partially hydrogenated oils have been used in most commercially prepared baked goods and for deep-frying in fast-food and other restaurants.

But there's a price to pay. The trans fat that ends up in partially hydrogenated oils boosts LDL (bad) cholesterol as much as saturated fat does. At the same time, it also depresses protective HDL (good) cholesterol. Trans fat has unhealthy effects on triglycerides, the main form of fat in the bloodstream. It makes blood more likely to form clots inside arteries, which can lead to a heart attack or stroke. It feeds inflammation, which plays key roles in the development of heart disease, stroke, and diabetes. By one estimate, getting rid of this bad fat could avert as many as 264,000 heart attacks, strokes, and other cardiovascular events each year in the United States alone.

Trans fat even throws a monkey wrench into ovulation and conception. The more trans fat in the diet, the greater the chances of ovulatory infertility.

There isn't a safe level of daily trans fat intake. The latest Dietary Guidelines for Americans recommends getting no more than two grams per day. Aiming for zero is even better. Avoiding trans fat takes some detective work, as we explain in Chapter 5.

In with the Good, Out with the Bad

Embrace the positive—include healthy fats in your diet and feel great about it. Your choices are varied and tasty, from pungent olive oil to creamy avocados and crunchy walnuts. Olive oil is an excellent source of monounsaturated fats. Use it to sauté vegetables, chicken, or fish; drizzle it over steamed vegetables; make your own mayonnaise, sauces, or salad dressings; even dip bread in it at the table. Canola oil, peanut oil, avocados, walnuts, peanuts, and most other nuts are other good sources of monounsaturated fats. To get more polyunsaturated fats in your diet, use vegetable oils such as corn and soybean oil for cooking and in salad dressings. Fish, soybeans, and soy products are other good sources, as are flax-, sunflower, and sesame seeds.

At the same time, cut back on saturated fats. Eating less red meat is one good way to do this. As we describe in Chapter 6, swapping meat for fish or beans has fertility-boosting benefits, too. Dairy products are another common source of saturated fats. Switching to skim or low-fat milk is ordinarily another way to edge excess saturated fats out of your diet. But that isn't such a good strategy for getting pregnant. Chapter 7 offers some startling evidence that a daily serving or two of full-fat milk or other dairy products may actually improve fertility.

Finally, avoid trans fats whenever and wherever you can. They do absolutely nothing good for your body or your chances of getting pregnant.

▶ Power Through Protein

Protein from meat, beans, eggs, milk, nuts, and other sources provides the raw materials for your body to build its own proteins and maintain the immune system. Protein can also be burned for energy or converted into blood sugar. The body doesn't store protein as it does fat or sugar, so you need to average about seven grams a day for every twenty pounds of body weight. It's a snap to get this much protein, and most Americans exceed this target.

Dietary protein does more, of course, than just provide building blocks and energy. Eating protein in place of easily digested carbohydrates may help prevent high blood pressure, heart disease, and some types of cancer. It may also be a good strategy for losing weight, something we talk more about in Chapter 10.

Research from the Nurses' Health Study, from a companion study being conducted in male health professionals, and from several long-term international studies suggests that the protein "package" matters and that protein from plants may be more healthful than protein from animals. That doesn't mean you should abandon meat and become a vegetarian. Instead, it calls for a "flexitarian" approach. This means relying more heavily on plant-based protein (beans, nuts, seeds, tofu, and whole grains) while also making healthful picks from the animal realm (fish, chicken, and eggs).

▶ Drink to Your Health

Beverages have traditionally taken a backseat to foods in nutrition research. Stay properly hydrated, so the thinking went, and what you drink to get there doesn't really matter. As with so many other nutrition myths, that one is giving way to the growing realization that what, and how much, you drink affects your health.

Early humans relied on one beverage—water. They also got fluids from their food, especially fruits and vegetables. Milk entered the picture with the domestication of animals. The advent of agriculture brought the pleasures of beer, wine, juice, tea, and coffee. The newcomers—soft drinks, energy drinks, and the rest—haven't been as welcome an addition.

Beverages replenish water lost through breathing, sweating, and urinating away metabolic wastes. If water out exceeds water in, minor dehydration ensues. It can make you feel grumpy and tired or can dull your concentration. Over the long term, chronic minor dehydration can cause dry skin, can contribute to constipation, and may lead to kidney stones or bladder cancer.

For simply replacing body fluid, almost any beverage will do. Water is best. It supplies everything you need without any calories and at little cost. Several glasses of water a day make an excellent start to staying hydrated. Have water with each meal and a glass of it in between meals. Add in some coffee or tea, if you want, and maybe a glass of wine for pleasure and possibly some extra health benefits. Go easy on the sodas, juices, and other sweetened beverages to avoid carbohydrate overload and gaining weight. If plain water doesn't appeal to you, try club soda, mineral water, or other fizzy water. If that's still too boring, add a slice of lemon, a wedge of lime, or a splash of juice. The goal is to get more water with fewer calories.

▶To Fertility and Beyond

The eating strategies we describe in this chapter embody the best science available on links between diet and health. They are good for women and men. They work for young adults, Generation Xers, baby boomers, and the oldest old. Along with exercise and not smoking, they are your best bet for warding off heart disease, cancer, diabetes, and a host of other chronic conditions. In the following chapters, we show you how these strategies, with a little tweaking, may also help you get pregnant.

Chapter 4

Slow Carbs, Not Low Carbs

KEY STRATEGY

Emphasize slowly digested carbohydrates over highly refined ones—beans, whole fruits, vegetables, and whole grains instead of white rice, white bread, and potatoes; avoid sugared sodas; go easy on juice.

O nce upon a time, and not that long ago, carbohydrates were the go-to gang for taste, comfort, convenience, and energy. Bread, pasta, rice, potatoes—these were the highly recommended, base-of-the-food-pyramid foods that supplied us with half or more of our calories. Then in rumbled the Atkins and South Beach diets. In a scene out of George Orwell's *1984*, good became bad almost overnight as the two weight-loss juggernauts turned carbohydrates into dietary demons, vilifying them as the source of big bellies and jiggling thighs. Following the no-carb gospel, millions of Americans spurned carbohydrates in hopes of shedding pounds. Food makers, spotting an incredible marketing opportunity, fashioned thousands of low-carb or no-carb foods; some even cashed in on the movement by slapping "no-carb" stickers on foods that never had any. At one point in the fall of 2003, plummeting bread sales prompted U.S. bakers to gather for a "bread summit" to talk about how the industry could rise to the Atkins challenge. Then, like all diet fads great and small, the no-carb craze lost its luster and faded from prominence.

It had a silver lining, though, and not just for those selling low-carb advice and products. All the attention made scientists and the rest of us more aware of carbohydrates and their role in a healthy diet. It spurred several solid head-to-head comparisons of low-carb and low-fat diets that have given us a better understanding of how carbohydrates affect weight and weight loss. The new work supports the growing realization that carbohydrate choices have a major impact—for better and for worse—on the risk for heart disease, stroke, type 2 diabetes, and digestive health.

New research from the Nurses' Health Study shows that carbohydrate choices also influence fertility. Eating lots of easily digested carbohydrates, such as white bread, potatoes, and sugared sodas, increases the odds that you'll find yourself struggling with ovulatory infertility. Choosing slowly digested carbohydrates that are rich in fiber can improve infertility. This lines up nicely with work showing that a diet rich in these slow carbs and fiber *before* pregnancy helps prevent gestational diabetes, a common and worrisome problem for pregnant women and their babies.[1]

What do carbohydrates have to do with ovulation and pregnancy? More than any other nutrient, carbohydrates determine your blood sugar and insulin levels. When these rise too high, as they do in millions of individuals with insulin resistance, they disrupt the finely tuned balance of hormones needed for reproduction. The ensuing hormonal changes throw ovulation off-kilter.

▶What Carbohydrates Do for You

It is lucky for us that we are not like cars, which can run on only one kind of fuel without major modifications to the engine. Instead, we can derive energy from any of the three major nutrient groups: fat, protein, and carbohydrate. That's because the body can convert carbohydrate and protein into blood sugar, which is formally known as glucose. Think of this six-carbon sugar as a kind of universal currency that cells of all types can then use for energy. Cells can also burn fat directly. Brain cells are particularly picky about their fuel and prefer having a supply of blood sugar—not too much, not too little—readily available.

Carbohydrates are the major component of breads, pastas, cereals, fruits, vegetables, and beans. They're the major contributor to blood sugar for the simple reason that all carbohydrates are made of sugar.

Anatomy of a Carbohydrate

Just three elements—carbon, hydrogen, and oxygen—make a dizzying array of carbohydrates. The simplest ones are single sugars like glucose, fructose (fruit sugar), galactose (part of milk sugar), and ribose (an important part of DNA). Because they contain only a single sugar building block, they are sometimes called monosaccharides. Next come the two-sugar carbohydrates, or disaccharides, which are made by joining two simple sugars. Table sugar (sucrose) is glucose plus fructose; milk sugar (lactose) is glucose plus galactose. After that come hundreds of carbohydrates made from sugars linked in more complex ways. These are generically called polysaccharides. The two most important polysaccharides are starch and fiber.

Starch is essentially a long chain of linked glucose molecules that our bodies can easily break apart. Fiber, on the other hand, is built in a way that withstands digestion and so passes largely unchanged through the digestive system.

Striptease

Throughout most of human history, the grains we ate came straight from the stalk. That means we got all of the goodness that grains pack in their three layers. Whole grains have a tough, fibrous outer layer called bran that protects the inside of the kernel. The interior contains mostly the starchy endosperm. Its job is to provide stored energy for the germ, the seed's reproductive kernel, which nestles inside the endosperm. The germ is rich in vitamins, minerals, and unsaturated oils.

When you eat unprocessed oats or whole barley, it takes a while for your stomach acid and digestive enzymes to break through the bran. Once they do, they are able to attack the starch and turn it into sugar.

WHAT ARE WHOLE GRAINS?

Whole grains are foods that contain all three parts of a grain's bounty: its fibrous bran, starchy endosperm, and vitamin-rich germ. Examples include whole or cracked wheat, oatmeal, brown rice, barley, popcorn, and an assortment of whole-grain breads, cereals, pastas, and crackers.

Processing completely changes the character and content of grains. Milling strips away the bran and germ, making the grain easier to chew, easier to digest, and easier to keep without refrigeration (the healthy oils in the germ can turn rancid, giving the grain an off taste). Refining wheat creates fluffy flour that makes light, airy breads and pastries. But removing the bran and germ strips away more than half of wheat's B vitamins and 70 percent of its iron (both of which are important for ovulation and conception, as we describe in Chapter 8), along with 90 percent of the vitamin E and virtually all of the fiber. Processing also pulverizes the starch, turning it from a small, solid nugget into millions of minuscule particles. Starch-digesting enzymes can break apart the fine particles in a flash, while it takes longer to disassemble the intact nugget.

Highly processed carbohydrates, such as white flour and cornflakes, give you a quick blast of blood sugar and only a shadow of the grain's original nutrients. Intact or minimally processed carbohydrates yield slower, lower, and steadier increases in blood sugar and insulin levels. They also deliver more fiber, vitamins, minerals, and other healthful nutrients.

▶Keeping Tabs on Blood Sugar

Cells throughout the body constantly need energy. That's why you have checks and balances that keep blood sugar levels fairly steady, even when you haven't eaten in a while. The exception is shortly after a meal or snack, when glucose levels rise temporarily. In general, this steady level, or safety zone, is between 70 milligrams of glucose per deciliter of blood (milligrams per deciliter is usually abbreviated as mg/dL) and 110 mg/dL. A deciliter is a tenth of a liter, or a little more than three ounces.

Two key hormones, insulin and glucagon, work together to get blood sugar into the safety zone after eating and to keep it there between meals. Both are made by the pancreas, a spongy organ the size and shape of a small banana that is connected to the small intestine. Insulin unlocks the molecular doors in a cell's membrane through which glucose must enter. Without insulin, cells have trouble absorbing this fuel even when they are bathed by it. (Brain cells are an exception—they can take up glucose without insulin's help.) Insulin also instructs the liver to process the glucose it sops up from the bloodstream into a starchlike substance called glycogen. The liver stores glycogen as part of the body's food pantry. Glucagon commands the liver to break down some glycogen and release it into the bloodstream. This helps maintain a steady supply of blood sugar.

Insulin and glucagon work together like this: Chomp on an ear of sweet corn and the digestive system turns the carbohydrates in the juicy kernels into sugar molecules. Glucose is shuttled into the bloodstream and whisked to the furthest corners of the circulatory system. The pancreas senses the rise in blood sugar and begins to churn out more insulin. Many hands make light work—the extra insulin helps muscle, fat, and liver cells efficiently absorb glucose. The movement of glucose into tissues drains it from the bloodstream. The pancreas responds to the decline in blood sugar by slowing its production of insulin and ramping up its secretion of glucagon. The liver responds to the extra glucagon by breaking apart some stored glycogen and releasing glucose into the bloodstream. This interplay of insulin and glucagon ensures that blood sugar levels stay in the safety zone.

Riding the Blood Sugar and Insulin Roller Coaster

Over the course of a day, the trajectory of your blood sugar and insulin looks like a roller-coaster ride. (See Figure 4.1.) The highs that follow meals and snacks turn to lows later on. Whether yours looks more like a kiddie coaster with gentle ups and downs or a hang-on-tight ride with steep climbs and breathtaking drops can make a difference to your

Figure 4.1 **Blood Sugar and Insulin Roller Coaster**

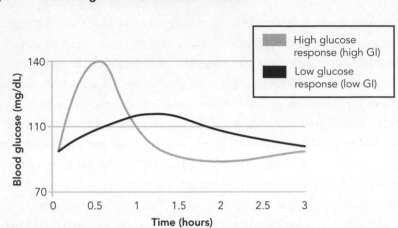

When you eat easily digested carbohydrates, your blood sugar and insulin levels rise quicker and higher and then fall faster and farther than when you eat slowly digested carbohydrates.

health and your fertility. No matter what your thrill-seeking sense, when it comes to blood sugar, take the kiddie coaster.

Eat a snack or meal brimming with easily digested carbohydrates— say, a baked potato or bowl of white rice—and your blood sugar skyrockets. The pancreas responds, as it should, with a big burst of insulin. But if that flood of insulin drives down glucose levels too fast, the pancreas may not be able to start making enough glucagon in time to stabilize blood sugar. Without help from the liver, blood sugar can cruise down to the edge of the safety zone and may even drop beyond it. Your gut and brain send out hunger signals that have you reaching for more food just as the liver starts releasing stored glucose. Blood sugar rises quickly once more, this time fed by food *and* a stream from the liver. The pancreas responds with more insulin, and . . . you get the picture. This cycle can leave you feeling hungry, even when you have taken in plenty of calories.

Sharp spikes and deep dips are one reason why eating a lot of the wrong kind of carbohydrates—those that the body almost instantly breaks down into sugar—can lead to weight gain. Acclimation is another, more dangerous problem, with repeated high spikes of blood sugar and insulin. Just as hardy Northerners get used to cold and snow, cells subjected to an endless bath of blood sugar and insulin get used to having a lot of insulin around and can eventually have trouble using only what used to be more normal amounts. Over time, the body needs more and more insulin to push the same amount of glucose into muscle and fat cells. This state of affairs is known as insulin resistance.

Abandoning carbs isn't the answer. By drastically cutting back on carbohydrates, you miss out on delicious and filling foods that give you fiber, vitamins, minerals, and a cornucopia of other healthful nutrients. Instead of no carbs, try slow carbs—whole grains, beans, fruits, and vegetables—that create slower, steadier changes in blood sugar and insulin.

Insulin Ignored

Resistance to insulin's "open up for sugar" signal is a sign of impending trouble. It's an early step on the road to type 2 diabetes (once called adult-onset, or non-insulin-dependent, diabetes). Insulin resistance is part of the metabolic syndrome, a constellation of problems that includes high blood pressure, excess weight, and high levels of triglycerides, the main form of fat in the bloodstream. These disorders often travel together and can add up to future heart disease. Insulin resistance is a hallmark of polycystic ovary syndrome, which affects millions of women. It also interferes with ovulation, making it a key player in ovulatory infertility.

When cells fail to heed insulin's signal, they absorb less blood sugar after a meal or snack. Glucose lingers in the bloodstream instead of gradually disappearing. The body responds to this situation in two ways. It immediately starts making more insulin. It's the same principle you might use when rearranging furniture—if a chair is too heavy for you to lift, you call in reinforcements. The extra insulin helps stuff glucose into cells. It also activates an alternate pathway for clearing blood sugar that involves turning glucose into fat and storing it in fat-storage cells called adipocytes.

In people who are resistant to insulin, this extra fat tends to accumulate in the midsection, wrapping around the heart, lungs, liver, and other organs. Fat that accumulates around the waist (technically called abdominal adiposity) may pose more of a health problem than fat around the hips and thighs—it has been linked with high blood pressure, high cholesterol, high blood sugar, and heart disease.

Everyone has high levels of blood sugar and insulin from time to time. Thanksgiving dinner or too many brownies in one sitting are enough to challenge the healthiest pancreas. This isn't a problem when it happens on rare occasions. Routinely high levels of blood sugar and insulin, though, wreak a slow, insidious havoc throughout the body. Over time, the overworked insulin-making cells in the pancreas begin to burn out and then fail altogether. This is the start of type 2 diabetes, a lifelong condition with no cure and numerous unfortunate consequences, from heart disease and kidney failure to blindness, loss of limbs, and premature death.

Not everyone who eats a lot of easily digested carbohydrates develops insulin resistance. It is, most likely, one of those problems that sit squarely at the crossroads of genetics and diet. People who inherit certain genes are more likely to develop insulin resistance. But over the past two or three decades, the human genome hasn't changed much while there has been an explosion in insulin resistance. Interactions between genes and diet or other lifestyle factors, especially the decline in physical activity, account for the bulk of insulin resistance. That's actually good news, because it means that almost everyone—even people who have many family members with diabetes—can take steps to guard against this health hazard.

▶ How Carbohydrates Affect Fertility

The single most common cause of infertility in women is polycystic ovary syndrome (PCOS). As many as five million American women have been diagnosed with this condition; many others have it but don't know it. PCOS can shut down ovarian function, often producing fluid-filled cysts on the outside of the ovary. (We described PCOS and its effects on fertility more fully in Chapter 2.) Many women with PCOS have insulin resistance, a breakdown in cells' ability to respond to insulin. The resulting high levels of blood sugar and insulin underlie many of the hormonal disturbances of PCOS. They have also been implicated in the infertility that routinely accompanies PCOS.

The problem of insulin resistance and high blood sugar isn't confined to women with this syndrome. A compelling study from Denmark published in 1999 showed that the combination can impair fertility in apparently healthy women, too. In this study, which included 165 couples planning to get pregnant, researchers looked at hemoglobin A_{1c}, also known as glycosylated hemoglobin, in the bloodstream. It is a measure of average blood sugar levels over the preceding three to four months. Women with high but still normal levels of hemoglobin A_{1c} were only half as likely to have gotten pregnant over the six-month study as those with low-normal levels.[2] Interestingly, women with high levels of hemoglobin A_{1c} had changes in their hormones and reproductive function that looked similar to PCOS but were not nearly as severe.

Findings from the Nurses' Health Study

Knowing that diet can strongly influence blood sugar and insulin, we wondered if carbohydrate choices could influence fertility in average, relatively healthy women. The answer from the Nurses' Health Study was yes.

We started, as usual, by grouping the study participants from low daily carbohydrate intake to high. One of the first things we noticed was a connection between high carbohydrate intake and healthy lifestyles. Women in the high-carb group, who got nearly 60 percent of their calories from carbs, ate less fat and animal protein, drank less alcohol and coffee, and consumed more plant protein and fiber than those in the low-carb group, who got 42 percent of calories from carbohydrates. Women in the top group also weighed less, weren't as likely to smoke, and were more physically active. This is a good sign that carbohydrates can be just fine for health, especially if you choose good ones.

The *total* amount of carbohydrate in the diet wasn't connected with ovulatory infertility. Women in the low-carb and high-carb groups were equally likely to have had fertility problems. That wasn't a complete surprise. As we described earlier, different carbohydrate sources can have different effects on blood sugar, insulin, and long-term health. Evaluating total carbohydrate intake can hide some important differences. So we looked at something called the glycemic load. This relatively new measure conveys information about both the amount of carbohydrate in the diet and how quickly it is turned to blood sugar. The higher the glycemic load, the more rapidly digestible carbohydrates are in the diet. (We describe glycemic load and its precursor, glycemic index, more fully later in this chapter.)

Women in the highest glycemic load category were 92 percent more likely to have had ovulatory infertility than women in the lowest category, after accounting for age, smoking, how much animal and vegetable protein they ate, and other factors that can also influence fertility.[3] In other words, eating a lot of easily digested carbohydrates increases the odds of ovulatory infertility, while eating more slow carbs decreases the odds.

Because the participants of the Nurses' Health Study complete reports every few years detailing their average daily diet, we were able to see if certain foods contributed to ovulatory infertility more than others. In general, cold breakfast cereals, white rice, and potatoes were linked with a higher risk of ovulatory infertility. Slow carbs, such as brown rice, pasta, and dark bread, were linked with greater success getting pregnant.

Computer models of the nurses' diets were also revealing. We electronically replaced different nutrients with carbohydrates. Most of these substitutions didn't make a difference. One, though, did. Adding more carbohydrates at the expense of naturally occurring fats predicted a decrease in fertility. This could very well mean that natural fats, especially unsaturated fats, improve ovulation when they replace easily digested carbohydrates, an effect we describe in Chapter 5.

In a nutshell, results from the Nurses' Health Study indicate that the *amount* of carbohydrates in the diet doesn't affect fertility, but the *quality* of those carbohydrates does. Eating a lot of rapidly digested carbohydrates that continually boost your blood sugar and insulin levels higher can lower your chances of getting pregnant. This is especially true if you are eating carbohydrates in place of healthful unsaturated fats. On the other hand, eating whole grains, beans, vegetables, and whole fruits—all of which are good sources of slowly digested carbohydrates—can improve ovulation and your chances of getting pregnant.

Bad Carbs Rule

The average American diet offers a truly frightening roller-coaster ride for blood sugar and insulin. Nationwide, carbohydrates contribute about 50 percent of all calories consumed.[4] A staggering half of those carbohydrate calories come from these eight sources, listed in descending order of their contribution:

- Soft drinks, sodas, and fruit-flavored drinks
- Cake, sweet rolls, doughnuts, and pastries
- Pizza
- Potato chips, corn chips, and popcorn
- White rice
- Bread, rolls, buns, English muffins, and bagels
- Beer
- French fries and frozen potatoes

Note that there isn't a fruit, vegetable, or bean on the list. Every item falls into the category of rapidly digested carbohydrate. They are made with either highly processed wheat or eminently digestible potatoes, or they contain plenty of sugar. With foods like these supplying half of our calories, it's no wonder we are in the midst of linked epidemics of obesity, insulin resistance, and type 2 diabetes.

A diet high in refined, quickly digested carbohydrates isn't so hot for the heart, either. It leads to higher levels of triglycerides, the main fat-carrying particle in the bloodstream, and lower levels of protective HDL cholesterol. Over time, these changes can damage the arteries and lead to a heart attack, a stroke, or other forms of cardiovascular disease. And it's a bust for fertility.

Smoothing Out the Curves

Not all carbohydrate-rich foods make blood sugar and insulin yo-yo wildly. Many have a slower, gentler effect. The problem is, you can't always tell which is which just by looking.

For years, scientists divided carbohydrates into two camps: simple and complex. Simple carbs were sugars like glucose and fructose, and complex carbs were chains of sugars, like starch and fiber. Nutrition guidelines urged us to eat complex carbohydrates instead of simple ones. The unspoken idea behind this recommendation was that simple sugars raise blood sugar faster and quicker than complex carbohydrates.

Measuring Up—Glycemic Index and Glycemic Load

The assumption that complex carbohydrates were better than simple ones went largely unchallenged until the 1980s, when a Canadian team made the bold move of actually testing it. They measured how several dozen carbohydrate-rich foods affected blood sugar levels in healthy volunteers. The results shattered long-held ideas that the body took longer to convert complex carbohydrates into blood sugar.

Nutrition scientist David Jenkins and his colleagues compared how fast and how high different foods boosted blood sugar compared to an equal amount of pure glucose. They called this ranking the glycemic index. Glucose was given a score of 100. The higher a food's glycemic index, the more it acted like pure glucose in the body.

Pure fructose (fruit sugar), among the simplest of simple carbohydrates, barely registered on the scale, with a glycemic index value of 20. This means that fructose generates just 20 percent of the blood sugar that an equal amount of glucose does. Cornflakes, cookies, and potatoes—complex carbohydrates by anyone's reckoning—raised blood sugar levels almost as much as pure glucose, as reflected in their glycemic indexes in the 90s.

Since the Jenkins team's first tests, the glycemic indexes of hundreds of foods have been measured. In general, a food with a glycemic index under 55 is considered to be a low glycemic index food, with a slow, steady effect on blood sugar and insulin. Medium glycemic index foods have scores between 56 and 69, while high glycemic foods weigh in at 70 or above. Table 4.1 lists the glycemic indexes and loads of several common foods.

The glycemic index is determined by comparing a volunteer's blood sugar response to fifty grams of pure glucose and then to an amount of the test food that delivers fifty grams of carbohydrate. Sometimes that leads to oddities. The glycemic index of carrots, for example, was originally calculated at a very high 92. But you have to eat one and a half pounds of carrots to get fifty grams of carbohydrate. A later modification, called the glycemic load, takes into consideration both a

Table 4.1 **Glycemic Index and Glycemic Loads of Common Foods**

Glycemic index and glycemic load offer information about how a food affects blood sugar and insulin. The lower the glycemic index or glycemic load, the smaller the impact on blood sugar and insulin levels. Low is considered a glycemic index under 55 or a glycemic load under 10. These values have been determined for almost 1,600 foods. Following are a few common examples. (A searchable database is available at www.glycemicindex.com.)

Food	Glycemic Index (glucose = 100)	Serving	Glycemic Load per Serving
Dates, dried	103	2 ounces	42
Macaroni and cheese	64	1 cup	32
Spaghetti, white	61	1 cup	27
Baked russet potato	85	1	26
Bagel, white, frozen	72	1 medium	25
Cranberry juice cocktail	68	8 ounces	24
Fruit Roll-Ups	99	1 roll	24
Fanta orange soft drink	68	1 can	23
Macaroni (plain)	42	1 cup	23
White rice	64	1 cup	23
Instant Cream of Wheat	74	1 cup	22

(continued)

Table 4.1 **Glycemic Index and Glycemic Loads of Common Foods**
   (continued)

Food	Glycemic Index (glucose = 100)	Serving	Glycemic Load per Serving
Pizza, plain dough with Parmesan cheese and tomato sauce	80	1 slice	22
Cornflakes	92	1 cup	23
Snickers candy bar	55	1 medium	19
Banana cake, made with sugar	47	3-ounce slice	18
Brown rice	55	1 cup	18
Corn chips, salted	63	2 ounces	17
Instant mashed potato	85	1 cup	17
Instant oatmeal	66	1 cup	17
Rice cake	78	1	17
Sweet corn on the cob	48	1 ear	17
Sweet potato	61	1 medium	17
Pretzels, oven-baked	83	1 ounce	16
Spaghetti, whole grain	37	1 cup	16
Baguette, white, plain	95	1 slice	15
Converted white rice	38	1 cup	14
Graham crackers	74	2	14
Whole wheat berries	41	2 ounces	14
Banana, ripe	51	1 medium	13
Black-eyed peas	42	1 cup	13
Oatmeal	58	1 cup	13
Orange juice	50	1 cup	13
Yam	37	1 medium	13
Bulgur	48	1 cup	12
Corn tortilla	52	1	12
50% cracked whole wheat bread	58	1 slice	12

Food	Glycemic Index (glucose = 100)	Serving	Glycemic Load per Serving
Kaiser roll	73	1	12
Navy beans	38	1 cup	12
Pearled barley	25	1 cup	11
Rye crisps	64	1 ounce	11
Honey	55	1 ounce	10
Pita bread	57	1 piece	10
Prunes	29	2 ounces	10
White bread	73	1 slice	10
Chickpeas, canned	42	1 cup	9
Ice cream, regular	61	½ cup	8
Grapes	46	4 ounces	8
Microwave popcorn, plain	72	1 ounce	8
Wheat tortilla	30	1	8
Baked beans	48	1 cup	7
Black beans	30	1 cup	7
100% whole-grain bread	51	1 slice	7
Reduced-fat yogurt with fruit	27	1 cup	7
Apple	38	1 medium	6
Pumpernickel bread	50	1 slice	6
Lentils	29	1 cup	5
Orange	42	1 medium	5
Tomato juice	38	1 cup	4
Cashews	22	2 ounces	3
Green peas	48	3 ounces	3
Milk, whole	27	1 cup	3
Peanuts	14	2 ounces	1
Hummus (chickpea salad dip)	6	1 ounce	0

Adapted from Foster-Powell K, Holt SHA, and Brand-Miller JC. International tables of glycemic index and glycemic load values: 2002. *American Journal of Clinical Nutrition* 2002; 62:5–56, and www.glycemicindex.com.

food's glycemic index and how much carbohydrate is in a normal serving. Calculating the glycemic load entails multiplying a food's glycemic index by the amount of carbohydrate in a single serving. For carrots, that would be 92 percent times six grams, or a value of about 5.

To make the concept of glycemic load easier to use, foods have been grouped into low, medium, and high categories. Foods with a score of 10 or less are low glycemic load, 11–19 is considered medium, and above 20 is considered high. So even though carrots have a high glycemic index, a single carrot has a small effect on blood sugar.

The most comprehensive list published to date appeared in the July 2002 issue of the *American Journal of Clinical Nutrition*.[5] It included almost 750 foods, ranging from angel food cake to yams. The University of Sydney in Australia maintains an updated searchable database at www.glycemicindex.com that now has almost 1,600 entries.

Focus on the Principle, Not the Numbers

Although the glycemic index and glycemic load are wonderful concepts, you don't need to eat by the numbers. Instead, following a few general principles can help you consistently choose foods with low, slow effects on blood sugar.

■ **Switch to whole grains.** Whole grains and foods made from them fall lower on the glycemic index than highly refined grains. A whole-grain breakfast cereal is an easy way to start the day and make the change to healthier carbohydrates.

■ **Don't pass on the pasta.** Pasta isn't the villain it's often made out to be. Most types have modest glycemic index values, although they have been stripped of their fiber and many vitamins and minerals. Whole-grain blends, which are now available in most grocery stores, are good, and real whole-grain pastas are even better. They're an excellent alternative to mashed potatoes or white rice, especially when tossed with olive oil and some Parmesan cheese.

■ **Bank on beans.** Beans generally have only a small effect on blood sugar and insulin. Equally important, including more beans and less meat in the diet is another way to improve fertility, as we describe in Chapter 6.

■ **Eat plenty of vegetables and whole fruits.** Vegetables and whole fruits (not fruit juices) have a low to modest effect on blood sugar and insulin. Like beans, they also deliver plenty of healthful nutrients. When planning meals and snacks, remember to think of potatoes as a refined starch, not a vegetable.

■ **Switch soda and juice for water.** Sugared sodas deliver empty calories—sugar without useful nutrients. They can be major contributors to daily glycemic load and seem to put a damper on fertility (see Chapter 9). Fruit juices, most of which are fruit-flavored sugar water, aren't much better. Calorie-free beverages such as water, sparkling water, and even sugar-free sodas are much better ways to slake your thirst.

■ **Don't sweat the small stuff.** Small differences in the glycemic index value and glycemic load don't matter much. Instead, try to choose foods with glycemic index values under 55 and glycemic loads in the low teens or below.

▶ Shifting to Slow Carbs

If you already eat carbohydrates that have kinder, gentler effects on blood sugar and insulin, congratulations. You have already broadened your culinary horizons, discovered great new tastes, and done your health, and fertility, a favor. If slow carbs are new to you, it is a snap to get one or more servings a day. Making the switch can improve the hormone cycles that guide ovulation. When you get pregnant, sticking with them is an important way to prevent gestational diabetes, a common problem that isn't good for mother or child. It can also help keep you from a later date with type 2 diabetes or heart disease.

Adding slow carbs to your diet isn't just about eating great grains, although that is an important part of it. Whole fruits, vegetables, beans, and nuts also deliver slow carbs. In general, most of them fall low on the glycemic index and glycemic load scales, meaning they have small, steady effects on blood sugar and insulin. The notable exceptions are potatoes, which can bump blood sugar into the stratosphere.

Combining slow carbs with healthful unsaturated fats offers a double benefit for fertility. Fats help slow the digestion of carbohydrates, which should help you feel full longer, a key element of weight control. Unsaturated fats also promote fertility, as we describe in Chapter 5, especially when you also cut out harmful trans fats. Good combinations include:

- Green beans with garlic sautéed in olive oil
- Hummus made with canola or olive oil
- Almond butter on whole wheat bread
- Wheat berries with chopped nuts and dried fruit

Finding Great Grains

Grains are the trickiest part of the slow-carb family. Some clearly fall in this group. Others can boost blood sugar as high and as fast as a drink of pure glucose. The difference is almost always one of processing. As a general rule, the more intact the grain, the lower the glycemic index. Sweet corn, for example, has a glycemic index of 48, while highly processed cornflakes have a glycemic index of 92.

Grains have nourished humans for millennia. Lately, though, we've lost touch with many of them. Few people venture much beyond wheat, rice, and oats. Try exploring the whole cornucopia of grains—it can add variety to your meals and years to your life. It includes barley, brown rice, bulgur (crushed wheat), kamut, millet, rye, spelt, teff, triticale, and wheat berries. Amaranth, buckwheat, and quinoa are used as grains, even though they aren't botanically grain plants. If you are unfamiliar with cooking grains, be sure to review Table 4.2, which offers basic cooking times and proportions. Books such as *The New Whole Grain Cookbook* by Robin Asbell and *Whole Grains Every Day, Every Way* by Lorna Sass contain a plethora of recipes and ideas.

Until recently, buying whole grains meant a trip to a health food store, specialty store, or co-op or ordering them through a catalog or online. Now mainstream grocery stores carry an array of whole grains, from breakfast aisles peppered with whole-grain cereals to whole wheat pastas and boxes of quinoa. Instant brown rice that cooks in fifteen minutes is available. You can even get whole-grain Chips Ahoy chocolate chip cookies, and Krispy Kreme has announced plans to sell a whole-grain, trans-free doughnut. We mention the latter two to make a point: just because something is made with whole grain doesn't make it a healthful food. It may contain a lot of sugar, salt, saturated fat, and other ingredients that don't measure up to the goodness

Table 4.2 **Grain Cooking Guide**

Whole grains usually take more water than the familiar 1:2 ratio of white rice to water. Some also take longer to cook.

Grain	Ratio of Uncooked Grain to Liquid (cups)	Cooking Time (minutes)
Amaranth*	1:3	20–30
Barley (pearled)	1:3	50–60
Brown rice	1:2½	35–45
Buckwheat groats*	1:3	15–20
Bulgur	1:2	5–20
Kamut berries	1:3	90
Millet	1:3	25–30
Oat groats	1:3	40–60
Quinoa*	1:3	15–20
Rye berries	1:3	40–60
Spelt berries	1:3	40–60
Teff berries	1:3	15–20
Triticale berries	1:3	40–60
Wheat berries	1:3	40–60
Wild rice	1:3	50–60

*Not technically grains, but can be used as grains.

of whole grains. Children's cereals often fall into this category, even though they are promoted as being made with whole grain. Consider the whole package when choosing what to eat.

Separating the Whole Wheat from the Chaff

Identifying whole grains is usually a cinch. Brown rice is a whole grain; white rice isn't. But what about foods made from grains? Does stone-ground wheat bread contain whole wheat or not? Sometimes it takes a bit of sleuthing. Food makers eager to jump on the whole-grain bandwagon have used a variety of labeling dodges to bamboozle consumers. These include terms such as *100% wheat, stone-ground,* or *organic* on food labels. None of these mean whole grain. The only foods that qualify are those with whole wheat, whole rye, or another whole grain as the first entry on the ingredients list. And even then the food could be made with a fair amount of enriched flour (which should really be called depleted flour, because only some of the nutrients that were stripped away in the refining process have been added back). Don't be fooled by the phrase *made with wheat flour,* as that's true of even the most highly refined white cake flour.

The new whole-grain stamp can simplify your search. It features a sheaf of grain on a golden background. Each stamp displays the number of grams of whole grain in a serving of food, as shown in Figure 4.2. All foods bearing the whole-grain stamp offer at least a half-serving (eight grams) or more of whole grain. Foods in which *all* the grains are whole grains—no refined grain is added—list "100%" on the stamp.

Adding Whole Grains

If you are new to whole grains, you can add a daily serving or more without too much ado. Here are some ways to add them to your meals and snacks:

■ **Breakfast.** The ready-to-eat cereal aisles of most grocery stores now stock many good whole-grain options. Choosing one or more of these can make a big difference. Cornflakes, for example, have a glycemic index of 92 and a glycemic load of 23, both very high values. Muesli has a glycemic index of 40 and a glycemic load of 6. If you favor

Figure 4.2 **Stamp of Approval for Whole Grains**

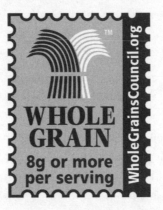

A growing number of whole-grain foods now carry a stamp like this showing the grams of whole grains in each serving.

Courtesy Oldways and the Whole Grains Council

hot cereals, trade your Cream of Wheat for oatmeal. If bread is what starts your day, try whole wheat toast, a whole wheat English muffin, or a whole-grain bagel. Keep in mind that most bagels contain enough carbohydrate to qualify as three or four servings. Whole grains are good, but too much of them can boost blood sugar as surely as refined grains.

■ **Lunch.** Have a sandwich on whole wheat bread or pack it in a whole wheat pita.

■ **Snack.** Reach for popcorn instead of potato chips. Whole-grain crackers dipped in hummus are an excellent hunger-busting option.

■ **Dinner.** If you like pasta, try one of the semolina/whole wheat blends now on the market, or go for a full whole-grain version. For a change of pace from rice or pasta, whole wheat couscous cooks in five minutes. Instant brown rice is ready in the time it takes to make white rice. If you're feeling adventurous, try cooking wheat berries, bulgur, quinoa, or wild rice.

You don't have to completely forsake white bread, white rice, or other processed grains. But the more you can make your grain choices whole rather than processed, the more you'll smooth out your blood sugar and insulin roller coaster. (For ideas, see Table 4.3.)

Slow Carbs for a Quicker Trip to Pregnancy

Quality, not quantity, is the key thing to remember about your carbohydrate choices. For fertility and long-term good health, go for whole grains, beans, vegetables, and whole fruits—foods that provide carbohydrates in slow-release packets along with a multitude of vita-

Table 4.3 **Making Smart Carb Choices**

For every meal and snack, there are slow-carb options you can choose instead of rapidly digested ones.

Instead of	Try
Soda crackers	Whole wheat crackers
Potatoes	Whole wheat pasta
Cornflakes	Total, Great Grains, or another whole-grain option
White rice	Brown rice or bulgur
Sugared soft drinks	Water, tea, sparkling water, diet soda, or milk
Cream of rice	Oatmeal
Candy bar	Fruit or nuts
Potato chips	Popcorn* or multigrain snacks such as SunChips
White bread	Whole wheat or other whole-grain bread
Fruit juice	Fresh fruit
Pretzels	Nuts
White potatoes	Yams

* If you are partial to microwave popcorn, make sure it isn't made with trans fats.

mins, minerals, and other phytonutrients. Eat them instead of refined starches, potatoes, sugar, sweetened sodas, and other foods and drinks that give you a quick blast of calories and little more. Making the switch to slow carbs can help you feel full longer after a meal or snack, which is great for controlling your weight and vital for controlling blood sugar. Such a switch will get you off the blood sugar roller coaster and maybe help put you behind the baby stroller.

Balancing Fats

In 2003, the government of Denmark made a bold decision that is helping protect its citizens from heart disease: it essentially banned trans fats in fast food, baked goods, and other commercially prepared foods. That move may have an unexpected effect—more little Danes. Exciting findings from the Nurses' Health Study indicate that trans fats are a powerful deterrent to ovulation and conception. Eating less of this artificial fat can improve fertility, and simultaneously adding in healthful unsaturated fats whenever possible can boost it even further.

How dietary fats affect fertility is a good fat–bad fat story, a mini-version of the fat saga that has confused our notions of healthful eating for some fifty years. Back in 1957, the American Heart Association's first attempt to come up with dietary strategies for preventing heart disease recommended eating more unsaturated (good) fat and less saturated (bad) fat.[1] It was a message far ahead of its time. Had we heeded it, countless people could have avoided heart attacks and strokes, and fewer lives would have been cut short by heart disease. Unfortunately, that prescient message was brushed aside by one that experts thought would be simpler, clearer, and easier to follow. Formally, the recommendation was "Reduce fat intake to under 20 percent of calories." What most people heard was "Fat is bad."

Many of us dutifully trimmed the fat from our food. Fats and oils, which once made up more than 40 percent of Americans' daily calories, now contribute about 33 percent. Guided by the low-fat mantra, we tossed out salad dressings and mayonnaise made with healthful olive oil or canola oil in favor of fat-free versions made with extra sugar. We replaced other fats in the diet with carbohydrates, usually the rapidly digested ones in white flour, potatoes, white rice, and sugar. This purge didn't make us any healthier. In fact, it may have contributed to the epidemic of obesity sweeping the country.

At the same time, we consumed stealthy artificial trans fats hidden in most commercially prepared baked goods and restaurant fried foods, blithely unaware of their presence or their hazards.

This combination—a move away from eating healthful unsaturated fats and consumption of trans fats—has had the disastrous effects of heart disease, diabetes, and other chronic conditions. Findings from the Nurses' Health Study indicate that this combo can also thwart efforts to have a child.[2]

▶The Skinny on Fats

The foods we eat contain four main types of fat: saturated, monounsaturated, polyunsaturated, and trans fats. Each one is made from a string of carbon atoms bonded to hydrogen atoms. What makes one fat different from another is the length and geometry of its carbon chain and how many hydrogen atoms it sports. Each fat family has its own characteristics and effects on health.

Three of these—saturated, monounsaturated, and polyunsaturated fat—should be part of every diet, though not necessarily in that order. The fourth, trans fat, is something you can, and should, live without. Table 5.1 lists common sources and recommended intakes of the four fat families.

Saturated Fat

Saturated fat gets its name from the fact that, in each member of this clan, every carbon atom is surrounded by the maximum number of

Table 5.1 **Types of Fats, Their Common Sources, and Recommended Daily Intakes**

	Fat Family	Good Sources	Daily Target
Emphasize	Mono-unsaturated fats	Olives and olive oils; canola, peanut, and other nut oils; hazelnuts, almonds, cashews, peanuts, and other nuts; peanut and other nut butters; avocados; sesame, pumpkin, and other seeds.	10 to 15 percent of calories* (22 to 27 grams)
Emphasize	Poly-unsaturated fats	Vegetable oils, especially corn, soybean, and safflower oils; soybeans and other legumes; walnuts; fatty fish such as tuna, salmon, herring, and anchovies. Foods that are good sources of monounsaturated fats also usually contain some polyunsaturated fats.	8 to 10 percent of calories* (17 to 22 grams)
Eat less	Saturated fats	Red meat; whole milk, cream, butter, cheese, and ice cream; coconuts and coconut products; palm oil.	Under 8 percent of calories* (under 17 grams)
Avoid completely	Trans fats	Any product containing partially hydrogenated vegetable oil. This includes many solid margarines; vegetable shortening; most commercial baked goods; and most fast foods. (Many products that once contained trans fats are now available in trans-free forms.)	Under 2 grams; zero, if possible

* For a diet of 2,000 calories a day.

hydrogen atoms it can hold. In chemical terms, the carbon atoms are saturated with hydrogen atoms. Saturated fats are straight chains, so they can pack together tightly. That's why they tend to be solid at room temperature (think of the congealed fat you see in a cooled pan of bacon grease). The foods we eat contain about two dozen kinds of saturated fat.

Foods rich in saturated fat include fatty meats such as prime rib, steak, sausage, corned beef, pastrami, bacon, and bologna, as well as the solidified animal fat known as lard. Dairy products such as whole milk, butter, and cheese pack substantial amounts of saturated fats. There are also a few plant-based sources, principally coconut oil and coconut milk, palm kernel oil, cocoa butter, and palm oil.

Your body needs some saturated fat. Eating it in moderation is fine (advice that can apply to almost all foods or nutrients). Go much beyond moderation, though, and you can run into trouble. Saturated fats certainly don't promote fertility. And over the long haul, the more saturated fat you eat, the more artery-clogging LDL cholesterol you have floating through your bloodstream and accumulating in patches inside your arteries.

Monounsaturated Fat

As the name implies, monounsaturated fats contain one special something that prevents carbons from pairing up with as many hydrogens as they can hold. That something is one double bond between two carbon atoms. This simple substitution gives monounsaturated fats the geometry of a bent stick. That shape prevents molecules from packing together, so monounsaturated fats are liquids at room temperature.

Good sources of monounsaturated fats are olive oil, peanut oil, and canola oil. Avocados, nuts such as cashews and almonds, and seeds such as sesame and pumpkin seeds are other excellent sources.

Eating monounsaturated fats in place of trans fats or carbohydrates provides a boost to fertility. These fats are also doubly good for the arteries—they tend to lower harmful LDL cholesterol and boost protective HDL cholesterol, an excellent combination. Monounsaturated fats also improve the body's sensitivity to insulin and ease inflammation.

Polyunsaturated Fat

The carbon chains in polyunsaturated fats hold two or more double bonds. They are even more crooked than their monounsaturated cousins and are also liquids at room temperature. The two most important families of polyunsaturated fat are the omega-3 fats and the omega-6 fats. (The names come from the position of the first carbon-to-carbon double bond in the fat's backbone.) Our bodies need polyunsaturated fats but can't make them, so we must get them from food.

Good sources of omega-3 polyunsaturated fats are fatty, cold-water fish such as sardines, salmon, and chunk light tuna. Because some types of fish contain high levels of mercury and other contaminants that can harm a developing child, it's important to choose wisely. For the best choices, see Chapter 6. Plant sources of omega-3 fats include flaxseed, walnuts, and canola oil. Eating soybeans or soy products and cooking with vegetable oils such as soy, corn, sunflower, and safflower oils provide both omega-3 and omega-6 fats.

Like monounsaturated fats, polyunsaturated fats are good for fertility. In the circulatory system, they lower levels of harmful LDL and increase protective HDL. They also do much more around the body. Omega-3 fats are an important part of cell membranes and so help regulate what goes in and out of cells. They provide the body with the raw material for hormones that regulate blood clotting, the contraction and relaxation of artery walls, and inflammation. They also help prevent the electrical impulses that give the heart its steady "beat now" signals from going awry.

Trans Fat

Saturated, monounsaturated, and polyunsaturated fats come from plants and animals. Most of the trans fats we eat come from industrial vats. They are by-products of a chemical reaction used to change liquid vegetable oil into a solid or to stabilize liquid oils so they won't spoil. Trans fats are such a potent deterrent to fertility, and are so bad for the heart and arteries, that we spotlight them later in this chapter.

Trans fats are found in hard margarines as well as many commercially made baked goods like cookies, crackers, and doughnuts. They

TRANS FAT LIMIT

The Dietary Guidelines for Americans and the Institute of Medicine recommend eating as little trans fat as possible. In practical terms, that means staying below two grams a day for someone who takes in two thousand calories a day. Going for zero is even better.

are also abundant in restaurant fried foods, especially fast foods. The average American eats about six grams of trans fat a day.[3]

Like saturated fats, trans fats increase harmful LDL. But they also decrease protective HDL, spur inflammation, and increase the tendency of blood to form clots inside blood vessels.

Fats Are a Potent Fertility Factor

Women, their midwives and doctors, and fertility researchers have known for ages that body fat and energy stores affect reproduction. Women who don't have enough stored energy to sustain a pregnancy often have trouble ovulating or stop menstruating altogether. Women who have too much stored energy often have difficulty conceiving for other reasons, many of which affect ovulation. These include insensitivity to the hormone insulin, an excess of male sex hormones, and overproduction of leptin, a hormone that helps the body keep tabs on body fat.

A related issue is whether *dietary* fats influence ovulation and reproduction. We were shocked to discover that this was largely uncharted territory. Until now, only a few studies have explored this connection. They focused mainly on the relationship between fat intake and characteristics of the menstrual cycle, such as cycle length and the duration of different phases of the cycle. In general, these studies suggest that more fat in the diet, and in some cases more saturated fat, improves the menstrual cycle. Most of these studies were very small and didn't account for total calories, physical activity, or other factors that also influence reproduction. None of them examined the effect of dietary fat on fertility.

The dearth of research in this area has been a gaping hole in nutrition research. If there is a link between fats in the diet and reproduction, then simple changes in food choices could offer delicious, easy, and inexpensive ways to improve fertility.

Connecting the Dots

The Nurses' Health Study research team looked for connections between dietary fats and fertility from a number of different angles.

Among the 18,555 women in the study, the total amount of fat in the diet wasn't connected with ovulatory infertility once weight, exercise, smoking, and other factors that can influence reproduction had been accounted for.[2] The same was true for cholesterol, saturated fat, and monounsaturated fat—none were linked with fertility or infertility. A high intake of polyunsaturated fat appeared to provide some protection against ovulatory infertility in women who also had high intakes of iron, but the effect wasn't strong enough to be sure exactly what role this healthy fat plays in fertility and infertility.

Trans fats were a different story. Across the board, the more trans fat in the diet, the greater the likelihood of developing ovulatory infertility. We saw an effect even at daily trans fat intakes of about four grams a day. That's less than the amount the average American gets each day.

Eating more trans fat usually means eating less of another type of fat or carbohydrates. Computer models of the nurses' diet patterns indicated that eating a modest amount of trans fat (2 percent of calories) in place of other, more healthful nutrients like polyunsaturated fat, monounsaturated fat, or carbohydrate would dramatically increase the risk of infertility, as shown in Table 5.2. To put this into perspective, for someone who eats two thousand calories a day, 2 percent of calories translates into about four grams of trans fat. That's the amount in two tablespoons of stick margarine, one medium order of fast-food French fries, or one doughnut.

What's the Fat-Fertility Connection?

Fats aren't merely inert carriers of calories or building blocks for hormones or cellular machinery. They sometimes have powerful biolog-

Table 5.2 **Relative Hazards of Trans Fat**

Eating trans fats instead of carbohydrates or more healthful fats significantly increases the risk of ovulatory infertility. Here's what we saw in the Nurses' Health Study:

Getting 2 Percent of Calories from Trans Fat Instead of 2 Percent from:	Increases the Risk of Ovulatory Infertility by:
Carbohydrates	73%
Polyunsaturated fat	79%
Monounsaturated fat	131%

ical effects, such as turning genes on or off, revving up or calming inflammation, and influencing cell function.

One example of this biological activity can be seen in polycystic ovary syndrome (PCOS), which we described in greater detail in Chapter 2. Women with this common condition are often overweight and have trouble becoming pregnant. They tend to be resistant to the action of insulin, a hormone that helps muscles and other tissues absorb sugar from the bloodstream. So they often have high blood sugar and are prone to developing diabetes. Drugs called thiazolidinediones improve the hormonal disturbances wrought by PCOS. These drugs, sold as pioglitazone (brand name, Actos) and rosiglitazone (brand name, Avandia), also improve ovulation and increase the odds that women with PCOS will have a successful pregnancy. Thiazolidinediones do this by latching onto tiny molecular triggers known as peroxisome proliferator-activated receptor gamma, or PPAR-gamma for short. The union of drug and PPAR-gamma activates a set of genes responsible for switching on insulin sensitivity in fat cells. This lets fat cells help clear sugar from the bloodstream after a snack or meal.

In other words, activating PPAR-gamma is a good thing.

Trans fats do just the opposite. They *quash* the activation of PPAR-gamma. The amount of trans fat in the average American's diet—about six grams a day—cuts PPAR-gamma activity in half. Shutting down PPAR-gamma means the body becomes *more* resistant to insulin. This, in turn, means higher blood sugar and insulin levels, which reduce fertility. At the same time, trans fats increase inflammation throughout the body, which interferes with ovulation, conception, and early embryonic development.

In contrast, unsaturated fats actually sensitize muscle and other tissues to insulin's "open up for sugar" signal. Linoleic acid, the most common polyunsaturated fat, does much the same thing as thiazolidinediones do—it activates PPAR-gamma, although it does so to a lesser extent.

In carefully controlled feeding studies, healthy people given unsaturated fats instead of saturated or trans fats develop greater sensitivity to insulin. The same thing happens in people with type 2 diabetes or those who are overweight. Other experiments show that eating unsaturated fats in place of saturated or trans fats decreases the body's production of glucose and appears to calm inflammation. The system-wide process of inflammation, so important for fighting infection and healing wounds, may also be at the root of heart disease, diabetes, and other chronic diseases. In short, unsaturated fats do things to improve fertility—increase insulin sensitivity and cool inflammation—that are the opposite of what trans fats do. That is probably why the largest decline in fertility among the nurses was seen when trans fats were eaten instead of monounsaturated fats.

▶ Eating for the Next Stage

If you are hoping to get pregnant, it's never too early to start eating as if you were. Adding unsaturated fats to your diet now, in addition to helping you become pregnant, may yield profound benefits for your child's mental and behavioral development. A new British study shows that children born to women who regularly ate seafood (the most important source of omega-3 fats) during pregnancy had better fine motor, social, and communication skills during their first four years of life.[4] At age seven, they had fewer behavioral problems than children of women who consumed little or no seafood during pregnancy. And by age eight, children of fish-eating moms were less likely to have below average performance on verbal and performance IQ tests.

Eating fish won't guarantee you a successful pregnancy or a smarter child. But these findings underscore a theme we touch on throughout the book: the tweaks or modifications the Fertility Diet recommends offer an opportunity to make healthy eating a lifelong habit, not just something to have a go at while trying to become pregnant.

▶Spotlight on Trans Fat

Think of trans fats as the evil cousins of the healthy omega-3 fats in fish, flaxseeds, and walnuts. The only natural sources of trans fat are bacteria living in the stomachs of cows, sheep, deer, and other ruminants. As a result, beef, lamb, buffalo, venison, and dairy products have small amounts of trans fat. Until a century ago, they were the *only* source of it.

Today, though, trans fats are everywhere, thanks to nineteenth-century chemists who discovered they could turn a liquid vegetable oil into a solid or semisolid by heating it and bubbling hydrogen gas through it. Oils that have undergone this process, known as partial hydrogenation, don't spoil or turn rancid as readily as nonhydrogenated oils. They can be heated to high temperatures again and again in restaurant deep fryers without breaking down. These characteristics have made partially hydrogenated vegetable oils a workhorse of the food industry. They are in stick margarines, vegetable shortening, packaged cookies and other baked goods, fast-food French fries and doughnuts, and scads of other foods. (See Table 5.3.) The FDA has estimated that until recently, 95 percent of prepared cookies, 100 percent of crackers, and 80 percent of frozen breakfast products contained partially hydrogenated fats. That means they also contain trans fats, inescapable by-products of partial hydrogenation.

Unlike unsaturated fats, trans fats aren't at all kind to your heart. Eating them boosts LDL, especially the small, dense LDL particles that are most damaging to arteries. It depresses HDL, which protects arteries by scavenging LDL from the bloodstream and artery walls and trucking it to the liver for disposal. Trans fats have unhealthy effects on triglycerides, the main fat-carrying particle in the bloodstream.

Table 5.3 **Amounts of Trans Fats in Some Common Foods**

This table lists the typical trans fat content of foods produced or prepared with partially hydrogenated vegetable oils. Now that food companies must list trans fat on food labels, many companies are removing trans fats from their products.

Type of Food	Grams of Trans Fat per Serving
Fast or Frozen Foods	
French fries	4.7–6.1
Breaded fish burger	5.6
Breaded chicken nuggets	5.0
French fries, frozen	2.8
Enchilada	2.1
Burrito	1.1
Pizza	1.1
Packaged Snacks	
Tortilla (corn) chips	1.6
Popcorn, microwave	1.2
Granola bar	1.0
Breakfast bar	0.6
Bakery Products	
Pie	3.9
Danish or sweet roll	3.3
Doughnuts	2.7
Cookies	1.8
Cake	1.7
Brownie	1.0
Muffin	0.7
Margarines	
Vegetable shortening	2.7
Hard (stick)	0.9–2.5
Soft (tub)	0.3–1.4
Other	
Pancake, from mix	3.1
Crackers	2.1

(continued)

Table 5.3 **Amounts of Trans Fats in Some Common Foods** *(continued)*

Type of Food	Grams of Trans Fat per Serving
Tortillas	0.5
Chocolate bar	0.2
Peanut butter	0.1

Values are from the USDA National Nutrient Database, the Harvard Food Composition Database, food packaging labels, and nutrition information posted by food makers.

They make blood platelets stickier than usual and so more likely to form artery-blocking clots in the heart, brain, and elsewhere. And they fuel inflammation, which plays key roles in the development of heart disease, stroke, and diabetes, and may also affect fertility.

Writing in the *New England Journal of Medicine*, one of us (Dr. Willett) estimated that eliminating industrially produced trans fat could prevent up to 264,000 heart attacks, strokes, and other cardiovascular events every year in the United States alone.[5]

The Institute of Medicine[6] and the USDA's Dietary Guidelines for Americans[7] recommend that trans fat intake be as low as possible. We believe that trans fats should be completely avoided—better yet, banned—just for the harm they wreak on the heart and circulatory system. Our findings that they also impair fertility, most likely by depressing or otherwise interfering with ovulation, is one more reason to expunge them from your diet.

Avoiding Trans Fats

For many years, trans fats were stealth fats, hidden in an array of foods and known only to savvy shoppers who knew the code phrases for them—"partially hydrogenated vegetable oil" and "vegetable shortening." That changed on January 1, 2006, with new regulations requiring food labels to list trans fat along with saturated and unsaturated fat, cholesterol, carbohydrate, protein, and the like (see Figure 5.1).[8]

That simple change is sparking a huge and healthy makeover of the American diet. Now that consumers can see which foods have trans

TRANS BAN

One way to take the guesswork out of avoiding trans fats is to ban them. Denmark did this in 2003. A year later, restaurants in the small town of Tiburon, California, voluntarily stopped using trans fats in their cooking oils, making it the first city in the United States to go "trans fat–free." But it wasn't until the New York City Board of Health required all restaurants to serve trans-free foods that the ban-trans movement really took off. That decision, in 2006, and the long planning that led up to it has roused other cities to action, or at least to discussion. Philadelphia instituted a trans ban, while Chicago, Boston, Washington State's King County, and other cities, counties, and states have been mulling such a move. These actions, though small, should hurry along food companies' efforts to find or adopt alternatives to partially hydrogenated vegetable oils. If a Burger King in Times Square can go trans-free, so can all the others around the country and the world.

The bans in New York City and elsewhere have had another equally important effect: they have gotten people talking about trans fats. The topic has been grist for Jay Leno's monologue, discussion on "Oprah," and even the subject of gentle ribbing on "Prairie Home Companion." Even if most governments decide to let the marketplace decide whether or not to ban trans fats, the ongoing discussion will help individuals be more aware of these harmful fats and steer clear of them.

fats and which don't, food companies are scrambling to remove trans fat from their products. "No trans fat" has become this year's "no cholesterol" or "zero carbs." Restaurants such as Legal Seafoods and Ruby Tuesday, which stopped using trans-rich partially hydrogenated oils long before it was fashionable to do so, have been joined by scores of others. Even before the 2006 label change, Frito-Lay switched to trans-free oils for making Doritos, Tostitos, Cheetos, and other snacks. The J. M. Smucker Company has created a Crisco with zero trans fat. Nabisco has spent millions of dollars developing a trans-free Oreo that tastes like the original. Hotels and food service companies are trum-

Figure 5.1 **Trans Fats Revealed**

Nutrition Facts

Serving Size 1 cup (228g)
Servings Per Container 2

Amount Per Serving

Calories 250	Calories from Fat 110

	% Daily Value*
Total Fat 12g	**18%**
Saturated Fat 3g	**15%**
Trans Fat 3g	
Cholesterol 30mg	**10%**
Sodium 470mg	**20%**
Total Carbohydrate 31g	**10%**
Dietary Fiber 0g	**0%**
Sugars 5g	
Protein 5g	

Vitamin A	4%
Vitamin C	2%
Calcium	20%
Iron	4%

*Percent Daily Values are based on a 2,000 calorie diet.
Your Daily Values may be higher or lower depending on
your calorie needs:

		Calories:	2,000	2,500
Total Fat	Less than		65g	80g
Sat Fat	Less than		20g	25g
Cholesterol	Less than		300mg	300mg
Sodium	Less than		2,400mg	2,400mg
Total Carbohydrate			300g	376g
Dietary Fiber			25g	30g

Before January 1, 2006, food labels didn't mention trans fat. The only way you could have known these harmful fats were in a particular food was to recognize the code phrases *partially hydrogenated vegetable oil* and *vegetable shortening* in the ingredient list. Thanks to a long-delayed FDA ruling, trans fat must now be listed. But there's a catch: a loophole in the labeling regulation lets food companies list zero trans fat on the label as long as the food contains less than 0.5 gram of it per serving.

peting their efforts to go trans-free and, of course, are using this as a marketing advantage. You can even take a trans-free cruise on the Royal Caribbean line.

Not all companies are moving so quickly. McDonald's, which pledged in 2003 to switch to nonhydrogenated oils, hasn't come through on that promise in the United States as of this writing. It is interesting to note, however, that McDonald's managed to go trans-free in Denmark when that country banned trans fats in 2003.

The new food labels haven't completely done away with the need to do some sleuthing. That's because a loophole in the labeling regulation lets food companies proclaim "no trans fat" on the package and list zero trans fat on the label as long as the food contains less than 0.5 gram of trans fat per serving. (In Canada, the cutoff is 0.2 gram per serving.) But five servings of "no trans fat" products that each contain 0.4 gram could push you right to the two-gram daily limit recommended by the FDA and Institute of Medicine.

Clearing trans fats from your diet still means squinting at food labels' fine print, where the ingredients are listed. If partially hydrogenated vegetable oil or vegetable shortening appears in the list, the food contains some trans fat. How much depends on what kind of oil was used and how much of it was hydrogenated, neither of which you can determine.

Restaurants aren't required to provide nutrition information about the food they serve, so getting trans fat information when dining out is still tricky. Avoiding deep-fried foods is one strategy, because many restaurants still use partially hydrogenated vegetable oils in their fryers. Some fast-food restaurants still serve up hefty doses of trans fat. At the time we wrote this book, in mid-2007, a 6-Strip Chicken Basket at Dairy Queen contained fifteen grams of trans fat. A KFC Chicken Pot Pie had fourteen grams. And a Sausage, Egg, and Cheese Biscuit with a large order of hash browns at Burger King set you back nineteen grams of trans fat, nearly ten times the daily healthy limit.

As the push to limit or phase out the use of partially hydrogenated oils takes hold in the food and restaurant industries, such fertility- and artery-damaging meals will, we hope, become a thing of the past.

When you go out to eat, don't hesitate to ask how a particular item is prepared. The more that servers and chefs hear this question, especially in regard to trans fat, the more likely that restaurants will switch to healthier oils.

▶Fats for Fertility

Unless you follow a low-fat diet, fats probably give you about one-third of your daily calories. Paying attention to the kinds of fats you eat and making smart choices can protect your heart and improve your overall health. Our findings from the Nurses' Health Study show that it can also enhance your fertility.

If choosing fats that can improve your chances of getting pregnant and your overall health were a dance, it would be a simple two-step:

1. Cut back on the fertility foe, trans fat.
2. Add in the fertility friends, mono- and polyunsaturated fats.

The cut-back part is old hat to most people raised with the old "fats are bad" dogma, while the add-in part may be a challenge—at least conceptually. In practice, though, it flings open the door to more flavorful foods and new tastes.

Don't drive yourself crazy constantly counting fat grams or computing percentage of calories from fat. You have better things to do with your time. What's more, there's no solid evidence so far that hitting specific goals for different types of fat makes a difference for fertility or good health. What is more helpful is getting to know what is in the foods you eat so you can make healthy choices.

Out with the Bad

To keep your weight stable, it's best to think about cutting back on unhealthful fats first. The most important part of this process is pruning trans fats from your diet. These mostly artificial fats depress ovulation and fertility and do nothing good for your arteries and the rest of you. As we described earlier in "Avoiding Trans Fats," this will take some vigilance.

■ **Read food labels.** Trans fats are now listed on the Nutrition Facts labels that grace most food packages. Due to a loophole in the labeling law, foods that contain up to 0.49 gram of trans fat per serving can indicate zero grams of trans fats on the label and proclaim "no trans fats" on the front of the package. So be on the lookout for the phrases that signal the presence of trans fats: "partially hydrogenated vegetable oil" and "vegetable shortening."

■ **When eating out, steer clear of fried foods.** Many restaurants and fast-food chains are still using partially hydrogenated oils to make French fries, doughnuts, and other fried foods. Some "white tablecloth" restaurants do, too. Ask your server if fried foods are prepared with partially hydrogenated oils.

■ **Don't bake with shortening.** Traditional solid shortening is chock-full of trans fat. When baking, try experimenting with liquid oils rich in unsaturated fats. If only a solid fat will do, trans-free Crisco and Spectrum Organic Shortening (from Spectrum Naturals, Inc.) are now available.

Moderation in the Middle

We don't lump saturated fats with trans fats because they aren't inherently "bad" like trans fats are. Solid studies have shown that eating some saturated fat is perfectly fine. Just don't overdo it. As a goal, saturated fats should account for no more than about 8 percent of your daily calories. If you usually take in two thousand calories a day, that's about seventeen grams of saturated fat. In practical terms, that's the amount of saturated fat in four ounces of milk chocolate, a fast-food cheeseburger, or a three-ounce sirloin steak.

Many people cut back on saturated fats by switching from whole milk to skim, giving up ice cream and sour cream, and eating no-fat yogurt. That's ordinarily an excellent place to start. But findings from the Nurses' Health Study indicate that one or two servings of whole-fat dairy foods actually improve fertility, as we describe in Chapter 7. Another prime source of saturated fats, red meat, appears to obstruct ovulation (see Chapter 6), so raising your meat consciousness can kill two birds with one stone. You needn't give up meat altogether. Instead:

- Have red meat once or twice a week instead of every night. In its place have fish or beans.
- Go for the leanest cuts available, and trim off excess fat.
- Keep serving sizes modest—no bigger than a deck of cards or the palm of your hand.

In with the Good

Here's the fun part. You can improve your fertility by adding healthful unsaturated fats to your diet. They are in a variety of delicious foods: olives, avocados, nuts, seeds, fish, beans, and many oils. There's no magic ratio of monounsaturated to polyunsaturated fats. Just include a mix of both.

- **Think in oils.** Olive oil and canola oil are excellent sources of unsaturated fats. Use them to sauté vegetables, eggs, and fish. Build your own salad dressings around them. Use olive oil in place of butter with dinner breads and rolls. If you love the taste of butter, try spiking your cooking oil with a bit of butter when sautéing. That way you get a buttery taste and the healthy goodness of vegetable oil. Experiment with oils from nuts and seeds, like almond, walnut, and sesame, for delicate flavors. Drizzle them on steamed vegetables or use them to dress salads.

- **Nut-ricious choices.** Contrary to popular opinion, nuts aren't junk food. They make for far healthier snacks than chips or candy. Try using nuts in main dishes, either as part of the sauce or in place of meat. Mediterranean and Asian cuisines use nuts this way all the time. Add nuts to salads, or sprinkle them onto sautéed vegetables for extra crunch and taste. In addition to peanut butter, try almond, cashew, and other nut butters for lunch, snacks, and sauces.

- **Omegas are for beginnings.** Your body can't make the poly-unsaturated fats known as omega-3 and omega-6 fats even though it absolutely needs them. Most people do a pretty good job getting all the omega-6 fats they need but come up short on omega-3s. Try to eat one or more good sources of omega-3 fats every day. These include fish, especially fatty fish like salmon, sardines, and chunk light tuna; walnuts; ground flaxseeds or flaxseed oil; and unhydrogenated soybean oil or canola oil.

No Fear of Fats

Just because a connection exists between trans fat and ovulatory infertility in the Nurses' Health Study doesn't mean it is the last word on the subject. It's actually just the first. This work needs to be corroborated, and we hope it will spur other research teams to tackle the issue in large groups of couples who are planning a pregnancy.

Yet there is no reason to wait for confirmation before showing trans fats the door. They do absolutely nothing good for you. You don't choose to eat trans fats; they are slipped into your food by food companies and restaurants. While partially hydrogenated oils rich in trans fat simplify life for the food industry, they only make yours more complicated and unhealthy. Trans fats are bad for your heart, arteries, and the rest of you. The more you eat, the greater your chances of developing heart disease, type 2 diabetes, dementia, or gallstones.

The finding from the Nurses' Health Study that eating trans fats also derails ovulation and prevents pregnancy is one more reason to avoid it like the hazard it is.

But don't let the threat of trans fats prompt you to avoid all fat. If you haven't already embraced the true goodness of unsaturated fats, not to mention their versatility and great taste, try adding more of them to your diet. Improving your fat balancing act—a little more unsaturated fat, a little less saturated, and no trans—is good for your heart, brain, muscles, and long-term health. It can help kick-start ovulation. And it's great for the new life you hope to be carrying.

Plant Protein Rules

Emphasize vegetable sources of protein over animal sources.

A t the centerpiece of most dinner plates sits, to put it bluntly, a hunk of protein. Beef, chicken, and pork are Americans' favorites, trailed by fish. Beans lag far, far behind. (See Table 6.1.) That's too bad. Beans are an excellent source of protein and other needed nutrients, like fiber and many minerals. And by promoting the lowly bean from side dish to center stage and becoming more inventive with protein-rich nuts, you might find yourself eating for two. Findings from the Nurses' Health Study indicate that getting more protein from plants and less from animals is another big step toward walking away from ovulatory infertility.

Table 6.1 **Top Sources of Protein**

Food	Yearly Pounds per Person
Beef	63
Chicken	59
Pork	48
Fish	17
Beans	8

Source: U.S. Department of Agriculture, National Agriculture Statistics Service. *Agricultural Statistics 2006*. (United States Government Printing Office, Washington, D.C.: 2006).

For years the main question asked about protein was, How much is enough to meet the body's needs? At long last, nutrition scientists are probing other important aspects of protein: What's the optimal amount of protein for good health? Are all sources of protein equally healthful? Can high-protein diets help you lose weight faster or better than low-fat or high-carbohydrate diets? Will they help prevent diabetes and heart disease? Is too much protein bad for the bones and kidneys?

Some of the credit for turning the spotlight on protein goes to the late Dr. Robert Atkins, who plugged the diet that bore his name for more than two decades before it hit its tipping point and swept across the country, becoming one of the biggest diet fads ever. The popularity of the Atkins diet forced researchers to take a good, hard look at dietary protein. They've learned that the protein in food does more than just supply the body with the raw materials to make its own proteins. It influences the feeling of fullness after a snack or meal and alters levels of insulin and growth hormones. The discovery that animal protein (meat) affects health in different ways than plant protein (beans, nuts, seeds, and grains) adds another twist. All these influences and differences affect fertility as well as long-term health.

▶Protein 101

Your body fashions all the proteins it needs from just twenty or so building blocks called amino acids. By stringing them together like beads on a chain, it creates thousands of different kinds of protein. Some are short, straight strands. Others are long, intricately folded structures that make origami look simple. Protein provides the structure for most tissues and an untold number of biologically active molecules. It can also be converted to blood sugar and burned for energy.

Your skin and hair are mostly protein. So is the hemoglobin that carries oxygen to your tissues, the immunoglobulins that defend you against infection, and the enzymes that keep you active and alive. Take away the water from your body and protein accounts for about 75 percent of the weight of what's left.

The amino acids in our proteins aren't unique to humans. Instead, the same ones are used by all living things, from bacteria to bison. It's an economical arrangement. The protein you get from a fish fillet or handful of peanuts is broken down into amino acids, which are then rearranged into you.

The human body has backup systems for almost everything. Making protein is no exception. As a guard against amino acid shortfalls, it can create thirteen of them from scratch. This baker's dozen are called nonessential amino acids. The others, called essential amino acids, must come from food. The protein in beef, fish, dairy products, and other foods from animals contains all the amino acids your body needs. This is *complete* protein. Protein from beans, grains, and vegetables is often *incomplete*, meaning it lacks one or more essential amino acids. Combining incomplete proteins, either in the same meal or eating them over the course of a day, can give you all the essential amino acids you need. Some classic food pairs, such as rice and beans, peanut butter and bread, and tofu and brown rice, are perfectly complementary, with each supplying one or more amino acids the other lacks.

How Much Protein Do You Need?

From the horrors of famine and war and the antiseptic work of the laboratory comes the fact that it takes about seven grams of protein for every twenty pounds of body weight to keep a body running smoothly. For someone weighing 140 pounds, that's fifty grams of protein a day, or seventy grams for someone weighing 200 pounds.

Worldwide, millions of children and adults don't get nearly enough protein. This shortfall stunts growth, shrinks muscle tissue, weakens the immune system, damages the heart and lungs, and can lead to early death.

In developed countries, getting enough protein is so easy that many people far exceed the minimum daily target. Oatmeal with milk for breakfast, a peanut butter and jelly sandwich for lunch, salmon for dinner, and a scoop of ice cream for dessert adds up to more than seventy grams of protein. And that's not even what you would consider a high-protein diet!

Although nutrition scientists know the minimum amount of protein needed to keep the body running, they don't yet have a handle on the *optimal* amount of protein in the diet. Answers to three questions will help determine that.

■ **Do high-protein diets make it easier to control weight?** It looks like it. A handful of recent head-to-head trials pitting high-protein diets against low-fat and other more traditional diets suggest that a high-protein approach may work a bit faster and better. As we describe in Chapter 10, eating protein instead of refined starches can make you feel full longer, which is an important step toward eating less. The body also spends more energy digesting protein than it does digesting carbohydrates.

■ **Does eating more protein reduce the risk of developing heart disease, type 2 diabetes, or other chronic diseases?** Eating protein in place of easily digested starch improves blood levels of cholesterol, triglycerides, and other risk factors for heart disease. A number of long-term studies, including the Nurses' Health Study, have shown that higher-protein diets, especially those with more protein from plants, offer some protection against heart disease. Whether eating more protein can prevent diabetes, cancer, and other chronic conditions remains to be seen.

■ **Is there a safe upper limit for protein intake?** This is a big unknown. High-protein diets are probably safe for most people. Note the qualifiers: *probably* and *most*. We say probably because there aren't solid, multiyear studies to provide the foundation for a more definite statement. And we say most people because eating a lot of protein can be hard on the kidneys, which filter out and excrete unused nitrogen, a product of protein digestion. Healthy kidneys have no problem handling this extra work. But it may weaken kidneys that aren't in such good shape. The Centers for Disease Control and Prevention estimates that nearly one in six Americans has chronic kidney disease, and those with high blood pressure and diabetes are at risk for it. There is also a theoretical concern that eating too much protein could weaken bones. The digestion of protein releases acids. The body usually neutralizes these with ease using calcium and other buffering agents in the blood. Eating lots of protein takes lots of calcium. If there isn't enough readily available in the blood, the body pulls some from its calcium storehouse—bone. This *could* weaken bones, but whether or not it does remains to be seen.

If your kidneys work fine, then the possible benefits of a higher-protein diet outweigh the theoretical risks. The case for a higher-protein diet is even stronger if you aren't partial to carbohydrates or you think they make you gain weight too easily.

There's neither a magic target for protein intake nor a ceiling for it. Getting up to 25 percent of your calories from protein—125 grams for someone who eats about two thousand calories a day—is perfectly reasonable, and some people get more.

If you want to get more protein, pay attention to the package it comes in. Not the box or the plastic wrapper, but the other nutrients that come along with it. As we describe in "All Protein Isn't Alike" later in this chapter, the fats, fiber, hormones, and other compounds in high-protein foods can enhance, or offset, the benefits you might get from a protein-rich diet.

Dietary Protein and Health

Other than providing the body with the raw materials to build its own protein, relatively little is known about how protein in the diet affects health. The most important connection has to do with allergies. These irritating and sometimes life-threatening overreactions of the immune system are generally triggered by proteins in food and the environment. Pollen proteins cause the misery of hay fever; gluten, a protein in wheat, rye, and barley, can set off celiac disease (see Chapter 8);

proteins from peanuts or other tree nuts can spark anaphylaxis, a sudden, severe, and potentially deadly reaction that can involve the skin, digestive system, lungs and airways, and heart. These three are just the tip of the allergy iceberg.

Beyond allergies, how protein in the diet affects health and disease is largely uncharted territory. That is especially true for how it might influence reproduction.

Protein and Infertility

Scattered hints in the medical literature that protein in the diet may influence blood sugar, sensitivity to insulin, and the production of insulin-like growth factor-1—all of which play important roles in ovulation—prompted us to look at protein's impact on ovulatory infertility in the Nurses' Health Study.

We grouped the participants by their average daily protein intake. The lowest-protein group took in an average of 77 grams a day; the highest, an average of 115 grams. After factoring in smoking, fat intake, weight, and other things that can affect fertility, we found that women in the highest-protein group were 41 percent more likely to have reported problems with ovulatory infertility than women in the lowest-protein group.[1] When we looked at animal protein intake separately from plant protein, an interesting distinction appeared. Ovulatory infertility was 39 percent more likely in women with the highest intake of animal protein than in those with the lowest. The reverse was true for women with the highest intake of plant protein, who were substantially less likely to have had ovulatory infertility than women with the lowest plant protein intake.

That's the big picture. Computer models helped refine these relationships and put them in perspective. When total calories were kept constant:

- Adding one serving a day of red meat, chicken, or turkey predicted nearly a one-third increase in the risk of ovulatory infertility.

A PALM OF PROTEIN

What constitutes a serving of fish, chicken, beef, or beans? The simplest way to visualize it is to hold out your hand, palm up. One serving of protein fits neatly into your palm. A deck of cards is another good stand-in.

- Adding one serving a day of fish or eggs didn't influence ovulatory infertility.
- Adding one serving a day of beans, peas, tofu or soybeans, peanuts, or other nuts predicted modest protection against ovulatory infertility.

Eating more of one thing means eating less of another, if you want to keep your weight stable. We modeled the effect that juggling the proportions of protein and carbohydrate would have on fertility:

- **Adding animal protein instead of carbohydrate was related to a greater risk of ovulatory infertility.** Swapping twenty-five grams of animal protein for twenty-five grams of carbohydrates upped the risk by nearly 20 percent.

- **Adding plant protein instead of carbohydrates was related to a lower risk of ovulatory infertility.** Swapping twenty-five grams of plant protein for twenty-five grams of carbohydrates shrunk the risk by 43 percent.

- **Adding plant protein instead of animal protein was even more effective.** Replacing twenty-five grams of animal protein with twenty-five grams of plant protein was related to a 50 percent lower risk of ovulatory infertility.

These results point the way to another strategy for overcoming ovulatory infertility—eating more protein from plants and less from animals. They also add to the small but growing body of evidence that plant protein is somehow different from animal protein.

▶Beyond Reproduction

Our understanding of how protein in the diet affects health is still in its infancy. Early findings suggest that it may influence heart health and the development of diabetes. Protein may also be an important part of weight-loss strategies.

Heart Disease and Stroke

Only two large studies, the Nurses' Health Study[2] and the Iowa Women's Health Study[3], have looked at whether protein in the diet influences heart disease or stroke. Similar results emerged from both:

- Eating a lot of protein or a little didn't cause or quell cardiovascular disease.
- Eating protein instead of easily digested carbohydrates offered some protection against heart attack, stroke, or dying early from cardiovascular disease.

An intriguing finding from the Iowa study was that protein from plants had a different effect than protein from animals. Women who got much of their daily protein from beans, nuts, grains, vegetables, and fruits were less likely to have had heart attacks or strokes or to have died of cardiovascular disease than those who got most of their protein from meat. A similar thing was seen in the Nurses' Health Study.

Diabetes

Controversial research has implicated proteins in cow's milk as a possible cause of type 1 diabetes (once called juvenile, or insulin-dependent, diabetes). That is one of several reasons why cow's milk isn't recommended for infants.

Later in life, the *amount* of protein in the diet doesn't seem to have any effect on the development of type 2 (adult-onset) diabetes. The *source* of that protein might. In the Nurses' Health Study, women who ate one or more servings of red meat or processed meat a day developed type 2 diabetes more often than those who had fewer than two servings a week. The connection with processed meat was very strong. Nurses who said they ate hot dogs, bologna, bacon, or other processed meats five times a week were 40 to 50 percent more likely to develop diabetes than those who rarely ate processed meats.[4] Eating high-protein nuts, in contrast, lowered the risk of diabetes.[5] (See Figure 6.1.) A companion study in

Figure 6.1 **Protein Packages and Diabetes**

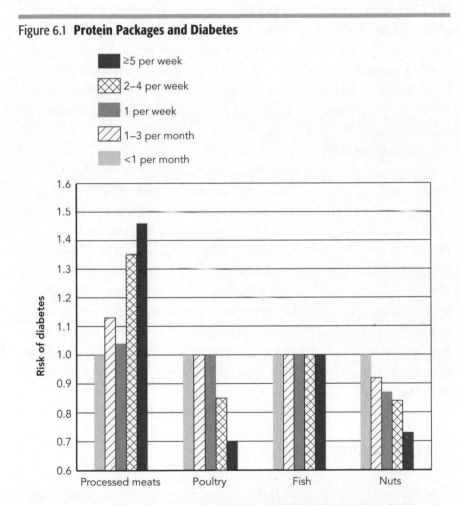

Other nutrients that come along with protein can influence its effect on health. In the Nurses' Health Study and a companion study in male health professionals, eating hot dogs, bologna, bacon, and other processed meats almost every day increased the chances of developing type 2 diabetes by nearly 50 percent, while frequently eating poultry or nuts decreased the risk.

men, the Health Professionals Follow-Up Study, showed the same noxious connection between processed meats and diabetes.[6] Later in this chapter, "Go Nuts" further explores the benefits of nuts.

Cancer

The role of dietary protein in the development of cancer is very much up in the air. Small studies have implicated eating a lot of protein in the formation or progression of prostate, colon, breast, and other cancers,[7] but this hasn't been borne out in long-term studies. It may not be protein in general, but protein from meat, that is the culprit. Several studies suggest that eating a lot of red meat is linked to the development of colon cancer and premenopausal breast cancer, while eating a lot of plant protein isn't.

Weight Control

The original Atkins diet touted a high-protein, low-carbohydrate, fats-be-damned approach as the one true way to lose weight. It isn't, of course. *Any* diet that helps you take in fewer calories will help you shed pounds. But a few head-to-head trials have shown that high-protein diets do help some people lose weight faster and more efficiently than low-fat, high-carbohydrates diets (see Chapter 10). Why? The body burns more calories digesting protein than it does digesting carbohydrates or fat.[8] Higher-protein meals suppress hunger and enhance the feeling of being full and satisfied longer than low-fat, high-carbohydrate meals and so help people eat less.[9] This may explain why high-protein diets help people lose weight faster and keep it off better than low-fat diets.[10]

All Protein Isn't Alike

If proteins were little more than strings of assembly-line amino acids that are interchangeable from species to species, then protein from animals and protein from plants should have identical effects in the body. But there is more to it than that. The body may respond to animal protein in different ways than it does to plant protein. It could be something in the proteins themselves, like a subtle difference between incomplete versus complete proteins. It is equally possible that the protein *package* is to blame.

Animal or Vegetable?

There's no simple answer to the question "Which is better for me, protein from animals or protein from plants?" Animal protein was long regarded as better because it is complete, meaning it supplies all the different types of amino acids that humans need. This eliminates the possibility of running short of one or more essential amino acids. But given the variety of foods available in many countries, even vegans—strict vegetarians who don't eat meat, fish, poultry, eggs, or dairy products—generally get all the amino acids they need.

A few old country-to-country comparisons of protein intake and disease show more heart disease in countries with more animal protein

EATING WITH THE ENVIRONMENT IN MIND

The question "Which is better for me, protein from animals or proteins from plants?" isn't limited to health. Some people make the choice based on environmental costs. According to the Union of Concerned Scientists, eating meat is the consumer activity with the second biggest impact on the environment, behind driving cars.[11] It takes twenty pounds of feed, mostly corn, to make one pound of edible beef. In comparison, we get one pound of chicken for every pound of feed. Raising cows, pigs, chickens, and even fish as agribusiness affects the environment in myriad ways, from water pollution to greenhouse gas emissions and global warming.[12] This isn't to say that growing plants is a purely "green" activity. Modern farmers use plenty of petroleum, fertilizers, herbicides, and pesticides to grow beans, grains, fruits, and vegetables.

Eating mostly plant-based foods won't wipe away the environmental impacts of food production. They will always be with us, in one form or another. But relying more on beans, grains, and other plants could ease the pressure on the environment today and in your children's future.

in the diet and less heart disease in countries with more vegetable protein. That's interesting, but it isn't proof that animal protein is bad for the heart. Exercise, smoking, and the amount of saturated fat in the diet, to name just a few other factors, also affect heart disease, making the country comparisons only a starting point for more research, nothing more.

Findings from other types of research, from long-term follow-up studies to short-term feeding experiments, support the notion that animal and vegetable protein somehow affect health in different ways.

The findings from the Nurses' Health Study and Iowa Women's Health Study on diabetes and heart disease described earlier support the idea that vegetable protein may do more than animal protein for good health and fertility. Small feeding studies have raised the possibility that eating soy protein provokes a smaller release of insulin into the bloodstream than does eating red meat or turkey. A study that included only women showed that higher intake of animal protein is related to higher levels of insulin-like growth factor-1; higher intake of vegetable protein isn't. While the body needs insulin and insulin-like growth factor-1, too much of them bog down ovulation. Excess insulin can increase the ovaries' production of male hormones, which can prevent follicles from maturing into eggs. High levels of these hormones can also decrease the body's production of sex hormone binding globulin, leading to higher levels of free—and active—testosterone throughout the body.

Together, this small body of work may explain why giving female pigs extra plant protein in the form of soybeans increases the number of eggs the sows release at ovulation. Similar experiments haven't yet been undertaken in women, but they should be.

Pay Attention to the Protein Package

Few foods deliver pure protein. Instead, it invariably comes with fat, carbohydrates, vitamins, minerals, and other nutrients. Some excellent sources of protein deliver decent doses of unsaturated fats, which are good for the heart, the brain, and other body systems. Other protein sources are chock-full of saturated fats, which aren't so good for the heart and blood vessels.

THE JOY OF SOY?

It has been hard to keep up with the fortunes of soy over the last decade or so. Headlines tell us that eating soy-based foods lowers cholesterol, chills hot flashes, prevents breast and prostate cancer, aids weight loss, and wards off osteoporosis. Soy products have flooded the market, expanding far beyond tofu and moving so far into the mainstream that soy milk has been advertised on the radio during Boston Red Sox games alongside doughnuts, oil additives, and beer. Yet the claims for soy exceed the evidence, and some studies warn that too much soy may increase the risk of breast cancer in some women or promote memory loss in others.

This doesn't mean you should turn up your nose at tofu or tempeh or ignore soy milk or edamame (a fancy name for soybeans). These foods are excellent sources of protein, calcium, and other healthful nutrients. Eat them in place of red meat and you are doing yourself a double favor. Just don't overdo it. Several servings a day is too much. Two to four a week is a more prudent target.

One reason for moderation is the estrogens that soybeans, and thus soy foods, contain. We don't yet know whether they suppress or promote breast or prostate cancer, help or hinder memory, and boost or blunt fertility. This uncertainty is the main reason why you shouldn't go overboard with soy and makes it doubly important that you not take tablets of concentrated soy or isoflavones extracted from soybeans.

Fats aren't the only part of the protein package to keep your eye on. Beans and nuts pack a variety of vitamins and minerals along with much-needed fiber. Dairy products are rich in calcium. Red meat delivers iron. Protein from soybeans and a few other plants contains estrogens that could be good for you. On the flip side, the heterocyclic amines created when meat is cooked to a well-done degree may be harmful, as may the nitrites and other preservatives in processed meats like hot dogs, bologna, and bacon.

The protein package almost certainly contributes to the health differences that are emerging between vegetable and animal protein.

If average consumption is any clue, then many Americans aren't very familiar with the bean, nut, and fish "packages." If you fall in that camp, what follows are some tips for adding more of them to your diet.

Go Nuts. If you think of nuts as just another junk food snack, you are missing out on a world of healthy flavors and foods. Nuts are a great source of protein and other nutritional goodies. One ounce of peanuts, walnuts, almonds, or pistachios gives you as much protein as a glass of whole milk, about eight grams. Nuts have more fat than milk, but these are mostly unsaturated fats that reduce harmful LDL cholesterol and boost protective HDL cholesterol.

One consistent, robust, and surprising finding from nutrition research is that eating nuts on most days of the week lowers the risk of heart attack or dying from heart disease by 30 percent to 50 percent. The evidence is strong enough that the FDA lets food companies claim on food labels that "eating 1.5 ounces per day of most nuts as part of a diet low in saturated fat and cholesterol may reduce the risk of heart disease." Nuts have a similar protective effect against type 2 diabetes and gallstones. In the Nurses' Health Study, the risk of developing type 2 diabetes was 21 percent lower in women who ate peanut butter five times a week than in women who rarely ate peanut butter. Eating whole nuts did the same thing.

With all the fat and calories packed into peanuts and other nuts, you might worry that eating them will expand your waistline. That's not necessarily the case. People who regularly eat nuts tend to weigh a bit less than those who don't eat nuts, maybe because nuts dampen hunger for longer than carbohydrate-rich snacks do.

You can't, of course, gobble nuts on top of your usual snacks and meals and expect to maintain your weight. At 160 calories per ounce, adding in nuts without cutting back on something else could translate into a ten-to-twenty-pound weight gain over the course of a year.

If you don't ordinarily eat nuts, an easy way to get more of this great source of plant protein is to have peanuts, almonds, walnuts, or other nuts as a snack instead of chips or a candy bar. After a bit, try using nuts instead of meat in main dishes. Mediterranean and Asian cuisines use nuts this way in all sorts of delicious dishes and sauces. Other tips for making your meals and snacks more *nut*-ricious include:

■ Top salads with pine nuts, pecans, walnuts, or another nut. Toasting them first for a few minutes gives them extra crunch.

- Add a handful of chopped nuts to hot cereal for extra flavor and a delightful crunch.
- Think nuts when you bake cookies, brownies, or other desserts.

Taking the Gas out of Beans. Beans are legendary for the flatulence they cause. Many people won't eat beans no matter how tasty and healthful they may be because of their gaseous aftereffects. The culprits are fiber and oligosaccharides (short chains of sugar molecules), both of which beans have in abundance. Fiber and oligosaccharides aren't fully digested in the stomach or small intestine, so they pass to the large intestine. Bacteria that call the colon home ferment fiber and oligosaccharides, giving off hydrogen, methane, and highly aromatic hydrogen sulfide gases in the process. They have to go somewhere and come out of you as flatulence.

Here are some tips to help you turn off the gas:

- **Start slow.** If you don't usually eat beans, start out with a small serving two or three times a week. As your body gets used to the fiber and oligosaccharides, you can gradually increase either the serving size or how often you eat beans.

- **Choose wisely.** Although there's little hard scientific evidence on this, some beans seem to create less gas than others. Those linked with little gas formation are adzuki and mung beans, lentils, and black-eyed, pigeon, and split peas. Heavy-duty gas formers include lima, pinto, navy, and whole soy beans.

- **Go soak your beans.** To get rid of oligosaccharides, and thus gas, the California Dry Bean Board advises soaking beans. In a large pot, add ten cups of water to one pound of beans. Heat to boiling, and let the beans boil for two to three minutes. Turn off the heat, cover the pot, and let the beans stand for at least one hour, though four hours or even overnight is better. During this soaking, oligosaccharides dissolve out of the beans and into the water. When you are ready to cook, *pour off the soaking water*, rinse, add clean water, and then cook as directed (www.calbeans.com/beanbasics.html).

■ **Add something to the pot.** Certain fruits, herbs, and spices are said to de-gas beans. These include papaya-based meat tenderizers, bay leaves, cumin, or kombu, a kind of seaweed. In Mexico, the herb epazote is prized for its gas-reducing abilities.

■ **Put your teeth to work.** The more thoroughly you chew beans, the more you expose them to natural oligosaccharide-digesting enzymes in your saliva.

■ **Bring on the Beano.** A few drops of this safe, natural enzyme product helps sensitive guts digest oligosaccharides. Sprinkle it on a bean dish or right on the tongue before your first bite of beans. You can find Beano in most grocery stores or pharmacies.

Fish When You're Eating for Two. Fish and shellfish are high in protein, low in saturated fat, and sometimes chock-full of healthful omega-3 fats. But there are contaminants to consider, too. Mercury accumulates in some species, while polychlorinated biphenyls (PCBs) can be found in others. Worries about mercury and other contaminants make some women shy away from eating fish. That's too bad, because the benefits of eating seafood far outweigh the risks for a woman and her current or future unborn children.

Mercury can cross from a mother to her developing baby via the placenta. High levels of it can cause brain damage. The effects of low levels are grist for great controversy. Some studies have demonstrated a connection between low mercury exposure in utero and later neurological and learning problems, while others haven't found ill effects. The effects of low levels of mercury in adults are speculative at best. What about PCBs and dioxins, which people tend to think of as powerful promoters of cancer? The Institute of Medicine calls the cancer risk linked to PCBs "overrated," because it was based on experiments in which animals were given huge doses for long periods. No one really knows if, or how much, cancer is caused by the low levels found in fish. What's more, most (91 percent) of the PCBs in the American diet come from beef, chicken, pork, dairy products, vegetables, and eggs.

Two large reports on the risks and benefits of eating fish, one from the Harvard School of Public Health[13] and one from the Institute of Medicine,[14] came to similar conclusions though from somewhat different directions: eating fish is worth whatever small risks the contaminants might entail. This holds even for, perhaps especially for, women planning a pregnancy or those who are already pregnant.

Omega-3 fats, such as those found in fish, are needed for brain development before and after birth. Small studies suggest that infants who get extra docosahexaenoic acid (DHA)—one of the two key omega-3 fats—have better mental and brain-body coordination. A large, long-term study of almost twelve thousand pregnant English women found that the children of those who ate less than twelve ounces of fish a week—the current U.S. recommendation for fish consumption during pregnancy—were more likely to score in the lowest quarter on verbal IQ tests.[15] They were also more likely to have problems with fine motor control, communication, and scores on social development tests. These results suggest that avoiding fish, which women often do because they are worried about mercury and other contaminants, doesn't protect babies from harm. What offers that protection is eating fish.

You can get the omega-3 fats you need, and that your baby will someday need, without harmful amounts of mercury and other contaminants by making smart choices. A good weekly target is to eat a five- to eight-ounce serving of fish two or three times a week.

■ **Maximize omega-3s.** When it comes to omega-3 fats, some fish are better than others. A three-ounce serving of farmed salmon contains 2,300 milligrams (mg) of omega-3 fats. Other omega-3-rich fish include herring, Atlantic mackerel, wild salmon, and sardines, with, respectively, 1,700 mg, 1,000 mg, 900 mg, and 840 mg per three-ounce serving. (See Figure 6.2.)

■ **Minimize mercury.** Small fish get mercury from eating algae and plankton. Bigger fish get it from eating smaller fish, and so on. With each step up the food chain, the mercury accumulates. Top predators, like golden bass (also known as tilefish), king mackerel, shark,

Figure 6.2 **Fish: Weighing the Benefits and Risks**

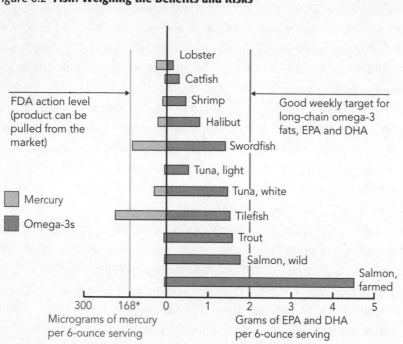

* Calculated from a limit of 1 microgram per gram (1 part per million).

Fish, shrimp, and other seafood are excellent sources of protein for general good health, for getting pregnant, and for nourishing a developing baby. Many of the benefits come from the omega-3 fats found in some species. Yet seafood can also contain mercury and other contaminants. Instead of steering clear of all seafood to avoid the small possible risk associated with mercury, choose types that contain little of it. If you are trying to get pregnant (or are pregnant or nursing a baby), don't eat king mackerel, tilefish (also known as golden bass), shark, or swordfish. Salmon and trout are good low-mercury sources of omega-3 fats.

Source: *Harvard Health Letter,* February 2007.

swordfish, and albacore tuna (white tuna), carry relatively high levels of mercury. These five are on the Environmental Protection Agency's (EPA's) advisory list for pregnant women. Freshwater fish can also accumulate high levels of mercury if the body of water in which they live is contaminated with the heavy metal. Notably, salmon has very low levels of mercury and plenty of omega-3 fatty acids. If you want to learn more about mercury in seafood, visit the EPA's website (www.epa.gov/waterscience/fish), which offers lists of low-mercury fish as well as state-by-state advisories for freshwater fish.

■ **Check the advisories.** Before eating fish that you catch, or those taken from rivers and small lakes, check the EPA's local fish advisories at the website listed above.

■ **Mix it up.** Because the levels of contaminants vary from species to species, one way to limit your exposure is to eat a variety of different fish and shellfish. Make sure you include salmon in the mix, as it is widely available and can be prepared in many delicious ways.

■ **Fish for the future.** If you are trying to get pregnant, go fish. Eating seafood is good for what you are trying to accomplish and, if you are successful, is even better for the new life you are starting.

▶Be Flexible

You need protein every day. Animal or vegetable? It's your choice. Possible health differences between the two in no way mean you are putting your health on the line by eating meat. But adopting a "flexitarian" approach to protein has long-term payoffs. This melds both the hunter and gatherer instincts still hardwired into our genes. Flexitarians focus on fruits, vegetables, grains, beans, and nuts but won't say no to poultry, seafood, or steak. In a nutshell, here's our flexitarian advice for general good health and fertility:

Get your daily protein from as many different sources as you can. Aim for at least half of your protein intake from plants—beans, nuts, peanut butter, whole grains, and seeds. Choose fish, eggs, and poultry for most of the rest, with less red meat and dairy products making up the balance.

To get the most out of your protein, pay attention to what comes along with it. If you are partial to beef, pork, or lamb, stick with the leanest cuts. Fish or poultry are better options. Plants usually provide the best packages.

If you are trying to work your way around ovulatory infertility, put plant protein to work for you. Add more beans, nuts, eggs, and fish. Let red meat be a treat instead of your daily fare. Skip bacon or sausages with breakfast. At lunch, have peanut butter and jam or egg salad on whole-grain bread instead of a roast beef sandwich on a deli roll. Snack on nuts instead of chips. For dinner, try black beans and rice with two vegetables or roasted salmon with a side of lentils and a salad with a sprinkling of toasted walnuts.

Chapter 7

Take a Break, Skim

KEY STRATEGY

Although a diet low in saturated fat offers many health benefits throughout life, a daily serving or two of whole milk or other full-fat dairy products may improve ovulation.

Consider the classic sundae: a scoop of creamy vanilla ice cream crisscrossed by rivulets of chocolate sauce, sprinkled with walnuts, and topped with a spritz of whipped cream. If you are having trouble getting pregnant, and ovulatory infertility is suspected, think of it as temporary health food. OK, maybe that's going a bit too far. But a fascinating finding from the Nurses' Health Study is that a daily serving or two of whole milk and foods made from whole milk—full-fat yogurt, cottage cheese, and, yes, even ice cream—seem to offer some protection against ovulatory infertility, while skim and low-fat milk do the opposite.

The results fly in the face of current standard nutrition advice. But they make sense when you consider what skim and low-fat milk do, and don't, contain. Removing fat from milk radically changes its balance of sex hormones in a way that could tip the scales against ovulation and conception. Proteins added to make skim and low-fat milk look and taste "creamier" push it even farther away.

▶Dairy—Demon or Delight?

Sometimes scientists follow a well-worn trail to new discoveries. Ours was just a few scattered bread crumbs. It would be an overstatement to say that there is a handful of research into possible links between consumption of dairy products and fertility. The vanishingly small body of work in this area is interesting, to say the least, given our fondness for milk, ice cream, and other dairy foods. The average American woman has about two servings of dairy products a day, short of the three servings a day the government's dietary guidelines would like her to have.

The dairy part of the Fertility Diet story starts with a hereditary disease known as galactosemia and a small survey of farm families in Wisconsin. Galactosemia is a relatively rare inherited disorder. People born with it can't fully digest lactose, the main sugar in milk. They have the enzyme needed to break lactose into its two component sugars, glucose and galactose. But their bodies can't convert galactose into glucose and use it for energy. Galactose builds up in the body. This can be deadly if not detected. Even when diagnosed and treated early with a lifelong, galactose-free diet, complications such as cataracts, liver degeneration, mental retardation, and tremors can still arise. Women with galactosemia begin menstruating later than normal, have great difficulty getting pregnant, and enter menopause early. These effects suggest that galactose is somehow toxic to the ovaries and raise the possibility that drinking milk might impair fertility.

Studies in animals support this idea. When female mice and rats are fed a very high galactose diet, they develop changes in their ovaries similar to those seen in women with galactosemia. The first study in humans, a country-to-country comparison of milk consumption, showed that fertility declined faster with age in countries where women drank a lot of milk than it did in countries where they drank little milk.[1]

Yet a survey of six hundred female farm workers in Wisconsin put a kink in the galactose-infertility connection. Women in the study who said they drank three glasses of milk a day were 70 percent *less* likely to have had problems getting pregnant than women who rarely drank milk.[2] That's just the opposite of what would be expected if normal amounts of galactose affected fertility.

Move Over, Skim

That work essentially formed the alpha and omega of research on dairy and fertility in humans when we began to look at possible connections between the two in the Nurses' Health Study. Because the work on galactose seemed to have a stronger biological foundation than the Wisconsin survey, our hypothesis was that women whose diets included several servings of dairy products a day would be more likely to have ovulatory infertility than women whose diets included little in the way of dairy products. That turned out to be wrong.

We first looked at total dairy intake. Nothing there. Nurses who reported having four or more servings of milk or other dairy foods a day were just as likely to develop ovulatory infertility as women who had one serving or fewer a week.

Lactose and galactose didn't make a difference. Women at the high end of the scale for both of these, whose daily dairy intake was the equivalent of three glasses of milk, had similar rates of ovulatory infertility as women at the low end of the scale. Calcium, vitamin D, and phosphorus, all important constituents of milk, didn't appear to affect fertility either.

What did make a difference was the *type* of dairy products the women in the study preferred:[3]

- The more low-fat dairy products in a woman's diet, the more likely she was to have had trouble getting pregnant.
- The more full-fat dairy products in a woman's diet, the less likely she was to have had problems getting pregnant.

It didn't take much to tip the balance toward or away from ovulatory infertility. One serving a day of a low- or no-fat dairy product increased the risk. One serving a day of a full-fat dairy product decreased it.

The depth and detail of the Nurses' Health Study database allowed us to see what foods had the biggest effects. The most potent fertility food from the dairy case was, by far, whole milk, followed by ice cream. Sherbet and frozen yogurt, followed by low-fat yogurt, topped the list as the biggest contributors to ovulatory infertility.

▶What's Going On?

How could something almost universally held up as a healthy food—skim or low-fat milk—contribute to ovulatory infertility while its full-fat relatives improve fertility? The answer to that question may lie in how skim and low-fat milk are made.

Taking Out

Milk straight from the cow contains 4 percent or more butterfat. The actual percentage depends on the breed of cow that made the milk, whether or not she was pregnant when giving milk, her feed, and the season.

Yet almost no one these days drinks milk with 4 percent fat. Even those who drink whole milk get a beverage that delivers a highly standardized 3.25 percent butterfat. Machines called separators are used to remove some or all of the fat from milk. Raw milk is piped into funnel-shaped stainless steel vats. The separators whirl these around about six thousand times a minute, creating a force several thousand times greater than gravity. The nonfat portion of milk, which is relatively dense, is pushed to the sides of the vats. Fat, being less dense (think of the old adage "Cream rises to the top"), collects in the center of the funnel. The fat is drawn off and packaged for other uses, like making premium ice cream, buttery pastries, and high-fat snack food. Separators can produce milk with virtually any fat content, from whole to skim. From there, the milk is pasteurized to destroy most of the microorganisms and homogenized to keep the fat that remains suspended in the milk instead of naturally separating from it.

Fat isn't the only thing the separators skim off. It turns out that some hormones are removed, too. This isn't as positive as it sounds.

Hormonal Changes. Although water, fat, protein, and carbohydrate (mainly lactose) make up the lion's share of milk, more than 250 chem-

NUMBERS GAME

Not that long ago, milk drinkers had three basic choices: whole, skim, or powdered. Look in the dairy case today and the options are almost overwhelming: whole, 2 percent, 1 percent, skim, reduced fat, fat free, no fat, less fat, and lactose free, not to mention the gaggle of flavored and vitamin-enhanced milks.

The proliferation of terms comes in part from an FDA ruling in 1998 that brought milk labels in line with those set for other foods.[4] Before then, 2 percent milk, which contains five grams of fat per serving, could be called low fat, even though the rules for other foods set the bar for low-fat foods at a maximum of three grams per serving. The milk industry was happy to oblige, because there was a concern that some consumers thought that skim milk had fewer nutrients than whole milk (the good stuff was "skimmed off" with the fat). Here's a quick guide to the terms:

- Whole milk contains 3.25 percent butterfat and eight grams of fat per serving.
- Two percent milk contains 2 percent butterfat and five grams of fat per serving. Two percent milk may not be called low fat. Instead, it is usually labeled as reduced fat or less fat.
- One percent milk contains 1 percent butterfat and 2.4 grams of fat per serving. It can be called low fat or little fat.
- Skim milk must contain under 0.5 percent butterfat, and usually has under 0.2 percent, making for a fraction of a gram of fat per serving. Skim milk is also called no-fat, zero-fat, or fat-free milk.

ical compounds have been identified in it.[5] These include vitamins, minerals, essential amino acids, hormones, growth factors, and a host of other substances. Some of them are dissolved in the watery part of milk; others attach themselves to fat particles.

The substances in milk with the greatest impact on fertility are hormones. Today's milk is a much richer stew of hormones than it was fifty years ago (see "Hormones in Milk"). Milk, cheese, and other dairy products contain female hormones such as prolactin, gonadotropin-releasing hormone, estrogens (estrone and estradiol), and progesterone. They also contain a batch of male sex hormones (androgens) or their precursors, including testosterone, androstenedione, dehydroepiandrosterone-sulfate, 5-alpha-androstanedione, 5-alpha-pregnanedione, and dihydrotestosterone.[5,6] Estrogens and other female hormones predominate, of course, since cows are females. (Although we follow convention here, calling estrogen a female hormone and testosterone a male hormone, keep in mind that women's bodies make testosterone and other androgens while men's bodies make estrogen.) Then there are the sex-neutral hormones, such as insulin-like growth factor-1.

Sex hormones like estrogen, progesterone, and some androgens are lipophilic (fat-loving) substances. In milk they are found attached to fat globules. Skimming off milk fat whisks away these hormones. Left behind in milk's watery part are some androgens, insulin-like growth factor-1, and prolactin. This shift doesn't bode well for ovulation.

An excess of male hormones unchecked by female hormones can prevent follicles from fully maturing. Extra insulin-like growth factor-1 can further widen the gap by depressing the body's production of sex hormone binding globulin. Because sex hormone binding globulin holds more testosterone than estrogen, reductions in it increase the ratio of testosterone to estrogen floating freely in the bloodstream. Too much prolactin, a growth hormone that stimulates breast tissue to make milk, can directly suppress ovulation, which is one reason why women usually don't get pregnant when they are breast-feeding.

The effect isn't entirely theoretical. An excess of androgens is a hallmark of polycystic ovary syndrome (see Chapter 2). In women with this condition, overproduction of male hormones contributes to their ovulatory problems and high rates of infertility.

Could male sex hormones from *outside* the body—say, from milk—have a similar effect? Concerned about this possibility, one of us (Dr. Willett) and several colleagues looked for an androgen-driven condition that could easily be measured. Acne filled the bill nicely. Excess testosterone is an important trigger for acne, and it doesn't take blood tests or fancy equipment to identify it. Exploring a possible connection between dairy intake and acne was a perfect project for a companion study of the Nurses' Health Study. Called the Growing Up Today Study,

HORMONES IN MILK

In 1900 the average cow produced about 3,000 pounds of milk a year. By 1950 that average was up to 5,300 pounds. Today it stands at 18,200 pounds, or nearly 2,100 gallons a year.[7] Some of this astounding increase is due to the commercialization and industrialization of the dairy industry. Dairy cows are no longer left on their own to forage in the open field. They are fed carefully prepared feed on precise schedules, and milking happens like clockwork. Some of the increase is due to selective breeding—mating cows that give more milk with bulls known to sire calves that grow up to be good milk producers. The genes that boost milk production are likely to be those for hormones such as insulin-like growth factor-1 and prolactin. The more potent or active these genes, the more the hormones they generate end up in milk.

In the past, on small family farms, cows were milked for about five months out of the year and, if they were pregnant, only during the early stages of pregnancy. On today's large dairy farms, cows are milked about three hundred days a year, and for much of that time they are pregnant. This keeps milk production high and allows a dairy farmer to keep making more cows without interrupting milk production. But it also adds extra hormones to milk. Milk from a cow in the late stage of pregnancy contains up to thirty-three times as much estrogen as milk from a nonpregnant cow.

One other hormone that deserves mention is bovine growth hormone, also called bovine somatotropin. It is normally produced by a cow's pituitary gland. Some dairy farmers inject their cows with a synthetic version to make them mature faster and produce more milk. This practice was met with a firestorm of opposition when it was first used in 1993. Critics charged that milk from cows injected with the hormone contained more insulin-like growth factor-1 than "regular milk." The controversy, along with high-profile public protests by Ben Cohen and Jerry Greenfield—aka ice cream maestros Ben and Jerry—put a damper on the use of bovine growth hormone. Today, only about one in ten U.S. cows gets injections of it. Extra insulin-like growth factor-1 is definitely a concern, but the contribution from bovine growth hormone is quite small compared to the contribution of milking pregnant cows.

it is composed of sixteen thousand children of women participating in the Nurses' Health Study.

In this group, acne was significantly more common in boys and girls who drank skim milk or low-fat milk or ate sherbet, cottage cheese, and other low-fat dairy products than it was in those who drank whole milk or consumed full-fat dairy foods.[6] This is the opposite of what you might expect if you think that pizza, chocolate, and other fatty foods lead to acne (which, by the way, weren't at all linked with acne in this study).

If drinking milk can affect the balance of sex hormones to the point that androgens are abundant enough, or strong enough, to stimulate the sebaceous glands in the skin (the source of acne), they could also affect the ovaries and other tissues.

Adding In

Remove fat from milk and that "creamy" taste gets lost. The color changes, too. Globules of butterfat are just large enough to scatter light, giving milk its characteristic white color. Without them, fat-free milk takes on a bluish tint. To cover up these undesirable changes, milk producers add in small amounts of protein extracted from whey, the liquid left over after all the milk solids have been removed.

Whey proteins aren't just inert additives. Instead, they have biological functions that could be directly involved in disrupting ovulation or conception. They may also act like miniature packhorses, lugging in other molecules that influence ovulation. One protein commonly added to milk is alpha-lactalbumin. Animals whose diets are enriched with alpha-lactalbumin become more energetic, gain more muscle, lose more body fat, and are more efficient exercisers than those fed diets enriched with whole milk.[6] These are classic effects of male hormones, suggesting that alpha-lactalbumin somehow has androgenic effects in the body.

▶ Dairy and General Health

Our recommendation to get one or two servings a day of whole milk or other full-fat dairy foods is a twist on the latest Dietary Guidelines for

Americans. They urge adults to get at least three servings a day of skim or low-fat milk or low- or no-fat yogurt, cheese, or other dairy products. The government's guidelines are bolstered by the slick, folksy milk mustache ads sponsored by the nation's milk processors. In these ads, popular culture icons like singers Beyoncé and Tina Knowles, soccer superstar David Beckham, figure skater Sasha Cohen, and actress Mariska Hargitay entice us to drink more milk.[8]

The government's guidelines aim to counter the calcium drain that is supposedly responsible for osteoporosis, the gradual loss of bone with age. (See Figure 7.1.) Fighting osteoporosis is a wonderful agenda. It affects more than ten million women and men in the United States alone.[9] Each year, osteoporosis causes 1.5 million fractures, including 300,000 broken hips. Hip fractures can be disabling and deadly. Almost a quarter of people who break a hip can no longer live independently and end up in a nursing home; another quarter die within a year.

But the strategy of more dairy products for all isn't the best way to fight osteoporosis. For starters, no one really knows how much calcium is needed to do the job. Even if we need the 1,000 to 1,200 mg of calcium a day that the Dietary Guidelines recommend for adults—

Figure 7.1 **A Dangerous Disappearing Act**

Normal, healthy bone

Osteoporotic bone

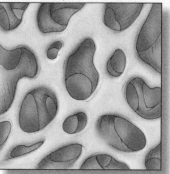
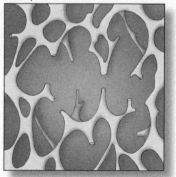

Under the microscope, healthy bone looks a bit like Swiss cheese. The tiny holes give bone incredible strength without being too heavy. Lack of exercise, too little calcium and vitamin D, smoking, and other hazards nudge the body to dissolve bone little by little. This loss of bone, known as osteoporosis, creates fragile bones that are prone to breaking.

CALCIUM ESSENTIALS

Your body contains about two pounds of calcium. Nearly 99 percent of it is in your bones. Think of calcium as the mortar that binds together and solidifies the bones' living tissue. The other 1 percent is dissolved in your bloodstream and the fluid inside your cells. Charged calcium particles help conduct nerve impulses, regulate your heartbeat, and control other cell functions.

which we probably don't—milk isn't the best way to get calcium. And the focus on dairy products and calcium takes the spotlight off other effective ways to keep bones strong and healthy.

Questions About Calcium

There is absolutely no question that healthy bones need calcium. This mineral is an essential part of bone, and its gradual loss can lead to broken hips, the tiny fractures that curve the spine and hunch over older people, and other life-changing problems. Almost every other big question about calcium, though, remains to be definitively answered.

How Much? The Dietary Guidelines gloss over the fierce scientific debate about how much calcium adults need each day. A look at recommendations from different countries highlights the controversy. Here in the United States, the guidelines call for 1,000 mg a day from ages nineteen to fifty and 1,200 mg a day after that. Canada sets the same goal of 1,000 mg for younger adults but boosts it to 1,500 mg a day after age fifty. In the United Kingdom, the target is half that: 700 mg a day for everyone over nineteen. The World Health Organization advises a comparatively paltry 400 to 500 mg a day. What's interesting is that each of these recommendations is based on the same body of evidence, none of which is compelling enough to lead to consensus.

If no one really knows how much calcium you need to protect your bones, why not play it safe and get as much as you can by drinking three glasses of milk a day? Because there are downsides to using dairy products to prevent osteoporosis. Millions of people can't digest milk, a problem called lactose intolerance. The fat and calories that

LACTOSE INTOLERANCE

Not everyone can digest milk. In fact, only a minority of the world's population has this dietary talent. A special enzyme called lactase is needed to digest milk. It cleaves milk sugar (lactose) into two simpler sugars, glucose and galactose. If the body doesn't make lactase, milk sugar remains intact. Lactose can't easily pass through the wall of the intestines into the bloodstream, so it remains in the intestines. Bacteria living in the gut jump on this wonderful energy source. One of the by-products is copious amounts of gas. This gas can cause stomach cramps, bloating, flatulence, and loose stools. This is called lactose intolerance.

Babies are born with the ability to make plenty of lactase. Most, though, stop making lactase between the ages of two and five. In some populations, especially those of northern European descent, people don't stop making lactase and can drink milk across the life span.

Worldwide, up to 75 percent of adults can't tolerate dairy products. In America, between thirty and fifty million people have trouble digesting lactose. Certain ethnic and racial populations are more affected than others. Up to 80 percent of African Americans, 80 to 100 percent of American Indians, and 90 to 100 percent of Asian Americans are lactose intolerant.[10]

come with the calcium are another. There is strong evidence that high intake of dairy products increases the risk of fatal prostate cancer and preliminary evidence that it also increases the risk of breast and ovarian cancers.

An ideal prevention strategy is one that stops something bad from happening without causing other bad things to happen. Getting a lot of calcium from dairy products to fight osteoporosis doesn't fit the bill.

What Else? It takes more than just calcium to make bone and keep it healthy. Exercise is at the top of the list. Bodybuilders and strength trainers know that the way to build muscle is to make it work. The same is true for bone. When you apply a modest force to bone by walking or with some other weight-bearing exercise, cells in and on it sense the physical strain. They respond with a flurry of activity that remodels the bone to make it denser and stronger. During childhood, exercise literally builds bone. During adulthood, it maintains bone health and limits bone loss.

Vitamin D is another important contributor to strong, healthy bones; it really should get at least equal billing with calcium. Vitamin D works in part by helping the digestive system efficiently absorb calcium and phosphorus. It actively inhibits the breakdown of bone and boosts the body's natural bone-building activity. Vitamin D deficiencies are common among older people with broken bones. In the Nurses' Health Study, older women who got at least 500 International Units (IU) of vitamin D a day were one-third less likely to have broken a hip than women who got less than 200 IU a day.

Few foods naturally contain vitamin D, so you need to get most of yours from sunlight or supplements. Going outside and letting the sun hit your face and arms for a few minutes a day gives you plenty of vitamin D. That doesn't work in the wintertime if you live north of a line connecting San Francisco, Denver, Indianapolis, and Philadelphia, where there is too little ultraviolet light to generate vitamin D. And many people can't, or don't, get outside every day. A more reliable way to get vitamin D is with a supplement.

The current recommendation for daily vitamin D intake is 200 IU (5 micrograms [mcg]) between the ages of nineteen and fifty, 400 IU (10 mcg) between the ages of fifty-one and seventy, and 600 IU (15 mcg) after age seventy. Those targets are probably too low. Many lines of evidence point to a higher level—at least 1,000 IU per day (25 mcg)—to get the full benefits of vitamin D.

Standard multivitamins carry 400 IU. Don't take two of these to get extra vitamin D, because that would give you a double dose of preformed vitamin A (retinol), which might counteract vitamin D's effects. Instead, try a standard multivitamin plus a calcium supplement that has added vitamin D, a good idea given that the two work better together than either alone. Or look for a supplement that contains 1,000 IU of vitamin D, which are now becoming available.

Vitamin K is a third nondairy strategy for building better bones. Found in green vegetables such as dark green lettuce, broccoli, and spinach, this vitamin helps regulate calcium in the blood. It is also involved in the formation and stabilization of bone. Women need at least 90 mcg of vitamin K a day; men, 120 mcg. Many people don't hit this daily target. An extra serving of lettuce or other green leafy vegetable each day can fix that.

Best Source? Milk is an excellent source of calcium. In the USDA's comprehensive list of calcium in common foods,[11] dairy products dominate the top fifty. A cup of plain, no-fat yogurt gives you 452 mg of calcium; a glass of whole milk, 276 mg. Milk is also brimming with fat, protein, carbohydrates, vitamins, and other minerals. No wonder it is a perfect food for fast-growing infants. But is it as perfect for adults who may be growing only around the midsection?

As you can see from Table 7.1, drinking three glasses of whole milk a day gives you 438 calories and 13.5 grams of saturated fat. That's the equivalent of a Big Mac and fries, or two-thirds of the recommended daily limit of 17 grams of saturated fat for someone on a diet of 2,000 calories a day.

The government's emphasis on skim or low-fat dairy products is one way to minimize the calories and fat that come with calcium. Even so, three glasses of skim milk a day give you 249 calories, along with a fair dose of hormones you can easily do without.

There are better ways to get your daily calcium. One option is turning to other calcium-rich foods such as spinach, black-eyed peas, canned salmon, or other foods listed in Table 7.2. An even simpler, virtually calorie-free option is taking a calcium and vitamin D supplement. A year's supply costs as little as $30.

▶ Practical Strategy

Our advice on milk and dairy products might be criticized as breaking the rules. The "rules," though, aren't based on solid science and may even fly in the face of the evidence. Long-term studies have consistently shown that women who drink a lot of milk or eat other dairy products aren't protected against fractures. And for solving the problem of ovulatory infertility, the rules may need tweaking.

Table 7.1 **The Skinny on Milk**

The big differences between whole milk and its lower-fat counterparts are in calories, total fat, and saturated fat. Here's what an eight-ounce glass of each contains.

Nutrient	Whole Milk	2% Milk	1% Milk	Skim Milk
Calories	146	122	102	83
Protein (grams)	7.9	8.1	8.2	8.6
Total fat (grams)	7.9	4.8	2.4	0.2
Saturated fat (grams)	4.5	3.1	1.6	0.13
Sugar (mainly lactose) (grams)	12.8	12.2	12.7	12.5
Calcium (mg)	276	285	290	306
Phosphorus (mg)	222	229	232	247
Potassium (mg)	349	366	366	382
Vitamin D (IU)	98	105	127	100

Source: U.S. Department of Agriculture National Nutrient Database for Standard Reference, Release 19 (2006).

Think about switching to full-fat milk or dairy products as a temporary nutrition therapy designed to improve your chances of becoming pregnant. If your efforts pay off, or if you stop trying to have a baby, then you may want to rethink dairy—especially whole milk and other full-fat dairy foods—altogether. Over the long haul, eating a lot of these isn't great for your heart, your blood vessels, or the rest of your body.

Before you sit down to a nightly carton of Häagen-Dazs ("*The Fertility Diet* said I needed ice cream, honey."), keep in mind that it doesn't take much in the way of full-fat dairy foods to measurably affect fertility. Among the women in the Nurses' Health Study, having just one serving a day of a full-fat dairy food, particularly milk, decreased the chances of having ovulatory infertility. The impact of ice cream was seen at two half-cup servings a week. If you eat ice cream at that rate, a pint should last about two weeks.

Equally important, you'll need to do some dietary readjusting to keep your calorie count and your waistline from expanding. Whole

Table 7.2 **Nondairy Sources of Calcium**

Dairy products are excellent sources of calcium, but they aren't the only good ones.

Food	Serving Size	Calcium per Serving (mg)
Ready-to-eat cereals	¾–1 cup	100–1,000
Collard greens, boiled	1 cup	357
Atlantic sardines, canned in oil	3 ounces	325
Spinach, boiled	1 cup	291
Green soybeans, boiled	1 cup	261
Turnip greens, frozen and boiled	1 cup	249
Yellow cornmeal, enriched	½ cup	241
Tostada with guacamole	1 tostada	211
Black-eyed peas, boiled	1 cup	211
Fast foods, taco salad	1½ cups	192
White beans, canned	1 cup	191
Pink salmon, canned	3 ounces	181
Kale, frozen and cooked	1 cup	179
Okra, boiled	1 cup	177
Dried soybeans, boiled	1 cup	175
Beet greens, boiled	1 cup	164
Tofu, firm (nigari)	¼ block	163
Corn bread (made with 2% milk)	1 piece	162
Trail mix with chocolate chips, salted nuts, and seeds	1 cup	159
Baked beans, canned	1 cup	149
Shrimp, canned	3 ounces	123
Ocean perch, baked or broiled	3 ounces	116
Halibut, baked or broiled	½ fillet	95
Peas, frozen and boiled	1 cup	94

Source: U.S. Department of Agriculture National Nutrient Database for Standard Reference, Release 19 (2006).

milk has nearly double the calories of skim milk, as shown in Table 7.1. If you have been following the U.S. government's poorly thought out recommendation and are drinking three glasses of milk a day, trading skim milk for whole means an extra 189 calories a day. That could translate into a weight gain of fifteen to twenty pounds over a year if you don't cut back somewhere else. Those extra pounds can edge aside any fertility benefits you might get from dairy foods. There's also the saturated fat to consider, an extra thirteen grams in three glasses of whole milk compared to skim, which would put you close to the healthy daily limit.

Aim for one to two servings of dairy products a day, both of them full fat. This can be as easy as having your breakfast cereal with whole milk and a slice of cheese at lunch or a cup of whole-milk yogurt for lunch and a half-cup of ice cream for dessert. Several of the recipes in Chapter 13 offer other ways to include whole milk or cheese in your diet. Easy targets for cutting back on calories and saturated fat are red and processed meats, along with foods made with fully or partially hydrogenated vegetable oils. Eating fish or beans or other plant proteins in place of hamburger, roast beef, pork chops, bologna, and other red meat would further help your efforts to improve ovulation and get pregnant, as described in Chapter 6. Reading food labels to spot products containing partially hydrogenated fats is a way to cut calories and avoid trans fats, which are a hazard for fertility (see Chapter 5).

Once you become pregnant, or if you decide to stop trying, going back to low-fat dairy products makes sense as a way to keep a lid on your intake of saturated fat and calories. You could also try some of the nondairy strategies for getting calcium and protecting your bones.

If you don't like milk or other dairy products, or they don't agree with your digestive system, don't force yourself to have them. There are many other things you can do to fight ovulatory infertility. This one is like dessert—enjoyable but optional.

Mighty Micros

D o you think of a daily multivitamin as insurance, a not-really-
necessary backup just in case your diet doesn't supply the
micronutrients you need? That's a decent definition for some
people. But for couples trying to get pregnant, a daily multivitamin
that delivers plenty of folic acid and iron can help. And it isn't just
for women—in addition to improving ovulation and other aspects of
fertility, a daily multivitamin can also improve sperm production and
quality.

A healthful diet generally delivers most of the micronutrients—vitamins and minerals—needed to keep the body's systems operating
smoothly. There are special situations, though, that demand more
than what food can provide. Older people who have trouble absorbing vitamin B_{12} need extra from pills. Food can't supply nearly enough
vitamin D for people who don't get out in the sun. Conception and pregnancy are two other scenarios. They require extra folic acid (one of the
B vitamins), iron, and some of the other ingredients in a multivitamin-
multimineral supplement.

It's almost always best to get your nutrients from food. But that can
be a tall order when it comes to folic acid and iron. Our findings from
the Nurses' Health Study indicate that at least 700 micrograms (mcg)
of folic acid are needed to improve ovulation and conception. That's
nearly double what is recommended for the average woman. For iron,

the fertility benefits begin to appear with between 40 and 80 milligrams (mg) a day, two to four times higher than the general recommendation for women.

A two-part strategy is the best way to hit these targets. Start with a healthful diet (see Chapter 3), and try to include foods rich in folic acid and iron. Then add in a multivitamin-multimineral supplement that contains folic acid and iron in the ranges that improve fertility.

Multivitamins

Up to half of Americans pop some kind of dietary supplement, usually a multivitamin pill, most days of the week. That's an incredible statistic when you realize just how little solid evidence there is to support this habit. Does a daily multivitamin prevent disease or help you live longer? No one really knows. It might. Then again, it might not—the issue is controversial.[1]

Preventing birth defects, though, is one area in which there is incontrovertible evidence that taking vitamins pays off. A daily multivitamin with extra folic acid dramatically reduces a woman's chances of having a baby with spina bifida, anencephaly, or another neural tube defect.

There is mounting evidence that vitamins also help couples trying to have a baby. An early hint of this came from one of the clinical trials that established folic acid supplements as a way to prevent neural tube defects. In this study, conducted in Hungary, nearly eight thousand women planning to have a child volunteered to start taking a supplement beginning a month before starting unprotected intercourse. Half of the women got a multivitamin-multimineral pill that contained substantial doses of twelve vitamins, including 800 mcg of folic acid, and seven minerals, including 60 mg of iron. The other half got an identical pill that contained just traces of copper, manganese, zinc, and vitamin C.[2] Neither the women nor their doctors knew who was getting which treatment.

Over the course of the study, the impact of folic acid was clear—zero neural tube defects occurred in children born to women taking the multivitamin-multimineral supplement, compared to six children born with the malformation to women taking the trace element pill. Overall, there were half as many congenital birth defects among children born to women taking the multivitamin.[3]

The Hungarian researchers didn't stop there. They checked to see if the multivitamin affected reproduction in other ways. It did. Menstrual cycles became more regular among women taking the multivitamin, while there was no change among those taking the trace element pill.[4] A slightly higher percentage of women taking the multivitamin (71.3 percent) became pregnant within a year than did those taking the trace element pill (67.9 percent).[3] And more twins were born to mothers taking the multivitamin.[5] Multivitamin use didn't influence miscarriage, preterm birth, birth weight, or the sex ratio.

Without corroborating evidence, the results from Hungary would be little more than an interesting footnote in medical research. That's because the trial wasn't designed to test whether a multivitamin affects menstrual cycles, conception rates, or twinning. However, other work supports the notion that a multivitamin can affect reproduction.

■ In Sweden, the National Board of Health determined that there were more twin pregnancies among women who took a multivitamin or folic acid supplement before conception than among those who didn't.[6]

■ University of Texas researchers found that the rate of twin births jumped in the state after the U.S. Food and Drug Administration started requiring food companies to add folic acid to grain products.[7]

■ A team from Boston University looked at data from five separate studies and found that mothers of twins were much more likely to have taken a multivitamin supplement than mothers of "singletons."[8]

■ A small, short-term pilot study tested a commercial supplement called FertilityBlend (containing chasteberry and green tea extracts, L-arginine, vitamins, and minerals) in thirty women who had been having trouble conceiving. Four women taking the supplement became pregnant compared to none taking a placebo. Although this could be due to the chasteberry, green tea, and L-arginine, the odds are just as good that the benefits came from the multivitamin component of the supplement.[9]

Taken together, this work suggests that *something* in a multivitamin enhances ovulation or the survival ability of embryos. In the twin studies, the "extra" twins were almost all dizygotic (fraternal) twins. Most dizygotic twins are the result of an additional egg being released during ovulation.

It is entirely possible that there's something other than the multivitamin at work here. In general, women who choose to take a multivitamin are a bit different from those who don't. They tend to smoke less, exercise more, and eat a more healthful diet; it could be these differences, and not the multivitamin, that account for changes in fertility. Yet most studies accounted for these differences using advanced statistical techniques and still saw a connection between multivitamin use and fertility. Equally important, some of the evidence comes from trials in which women were randomly assigned to take an unmarked pill, either a multivitamin or a placebo, and didn't learn until after the trial had ended which one they had been taking.

▶Lessons from the Nurses

This intriguing work sparked our interest in exploring connections between multivitamin use and ovulatory infertility in the Nurses' Health Study.

Almost 60 percent of the study participants reported taking multivitamins, significantly higher than the national average. That probably reflects the fact that many of these women were trying to get pregnant, and taking a multivitamin with folic acid is a standard recommendation for pregnancy planners.

As a group, the women who took multivitamins were 40 percent less likely to have encountered ovulatory infertility over an eight-year period than women who didn't take them.[10] Although these supplements contain a dozen or so ingredients, computer models suggested that just two—folic acid and iron—made the biggest contribution to this reduction.

So we looked at each of these separately. For folic acid, women who got at least 700 mcg a day from diet and supplements were 40 to 50 percent less likely to have had ovulatory infertility than women getting less than 300 mcg a day.

The results for iron were a bit more surprising. Women who regularly took an iron supplement were 40 percent less likely to have had trouble getting pregnant than women who didn't take iron. A little bit of iron didn't seem to have much of an effect—the benefit came with relatively high daily doses of 40 to 80 mg. What was unexpected was that the *source* of the iron mattered. Women who got most of their iron from meat (heme iron) weren't protected at all against ovulatory infertility, and there was a hint that high intake of iron from meat actually *increased* the chances of developing it. In contrast, iron from fruits, vegetables, beans, and supplements (nonheme iron) improved the chances of getting pregnant.[11]

How folic acid and iron help improve ovulation and conception probably has something to do with their roles at the nexus of cell division.

▶A Busy B

Once upon a time, folic acid was just an ordinary, hardworking vitamin, one of eight B vitamins that help a variety of enzymes do their jobs. The discovery of a direct link between a mother's low intake of folic acid and birth defects such as spina bifida and anencephaly put it in the spotlight. Hints that higher intake of folic acid may also protect against heart disease, stroke, and some types of cancer have further heightened its profile, although these connections have yet to be proved. And now there's a wave of research supporting folic acid as a fertility booster in women and men.

You might expect a dietary superstar like folic acid to do big things in the body. Yet its job is actually quite small and specific: it shuttles single carbon atoms bristling with hydrogens and oxygens from one

FOLIC ACID OR FOLATE?

The B vitamin we talk about in this chapter exists in several forms. *Folate* is the type that occurs naturally in food, circulates in the bloodstream, and is found inside red blood cells. *Folic acid* is a synthetic form of folate used in vitamin supplements and in fortifying foods.

Folic acid is easier for the body to assimilate than naturally occurring food folate. That's why the Institute of Medicine introduced a new unit— the Dietary Folate Equivalent (DFE)—when it set the latest recommendations for folate in 1998. Here is how they stack up:

- 1 mcg of natural food folate provides 1 mcg of DFE.
- 1 mcg of folic acid taken with meals or as part of a fortified food provides 1.7 mcg of DFE.
- 1 mcg of a folic acid supplement taken on an empty stomach provides 2 mcg of DFE.

chemical compound to another. That tiny transfer, though, puts folic acid at the innermost circle of life. It is a vital part of building DNA, the double helix that carries the body's operating manual. Folate-assisted transfers are also essential for converting some amino acids into others. Amino acids are building blocks the body uses to assemble the thousands of proteins it needs for everything from extracting energy from food to building skin, muscle, and other tissues. The ability to change one amino acid into another guarantees that the body has a steady supply of *all* amino acids, even when the diet is supplying too much of one kind and not enough of another.

Reproduction is a time of furious DNA replication and protein assembly. No wonder that folic acid appears to influence the start of a pregnancy or its continuation, as well as prevent birth defects. Like a small ship embarking on a difficult voyage, an embryo must survive on what it has stored or can pick up until it establishes connections with the mother's circulation. Having an adequate supply of folate in the bloodstream before conception ensures that the egg or embryo never runs low on this essential nutrient.

Extra folate may improve a woman's chances of getting pregnant and staying pregnant in several other ways as well. One has to do with its role in recycling homocysteine, a potentially toxic amino acid. Folate helps turn homocysteine into methionine, a benign amino acid that is intimately involved in regulating many genes. Too little folate can lead to a high level of homocysteine, which has been linked with heart disease, stroke, and rapid loss of memory or thinking skills with age. Homocysteine also appears to affect reproduction. Women with high homocysteine are more likely to have early miscarriages and severe high blood pressure during pregnancy (preeclampsia). Getting extra folate is one way to keep homocysteine levels low.

Taking folic acid may also somehow directly stimulate ovulation. In several trials, women taking folic acid supplements were more likely to spontaneously have fraternal twins than those taking a placebo. Fraternal twins come from the fertilization of two separate eggs, suggesting that folic acid promotes ovulation.

The data from the Nurses' Health Study isn't the only evidence that folate is intimately involved in ovulation. Hints from a serious digestive problem, animal studies, and assisted reproduction also point in that direction.

Clues from Sprue

Celiac disease, once called celiac sprue, is a serious digestive disorder. It is caused by the body's intolerance to gluten, a protein found in grains such as wheat, barley, and rye. In people with celiac disease, the gluten in just a few bites of bread can trigger an attack by the immune system. Instead of targeting only the gluten, white blood cells and other immune-system warriors also assault the small intestine. Over time, the cumulative damage from these attacks destroys the small intestine's ability to absorb vital nutrients from food. Key losses include folic acid, iron, and a host of other micronutrients. Once celiac disease is diagnosed—which often takes years—the main treatment is a strict gluten-free diet.

Women with undiagnosed or untreated celiac disease begin menstruating at a later age, start menopause earlier, are more likely to have irregular menstrual cycles, and often have trouble getting pregnant. In fact, undiagnosed celiac disease may account for up to 8 percent of all cases of so-called unexplained infertility. The trio of delayed menstruation, earlier menopause, and menstrual irregularities cast suspicion on ovulatory problems as the source of celiac-related infertility. In men, celiac disease can interfere with production of sex hormones and sperm.

Avoiding gluten sometimes leads to a return of fertility in both women and men. Yet infertility problems can linger even when celiac disease is completely under control with a gluten-free diet. It is possible that the immune-system derangement that causes the body to respond so violently to gluten somehow throws off reproductive hormones or affects reproduction in other ways. It is equally possible that deficiencies in folate, iron, vitamin D, vitamin K, and other micronutrients that accompany even well-controlled celiac disease are the culprit.

Nearly forty years ago, a British doctor wrote about a patient of his with celiac disease who had been unable to conceive for five years.[12] Because of a low blood level of folate, she started taking five grams (5,000 mcg) of folic acid a day in May of 1968. By July she was pregnant, and she delivered a healthy baby the following March. She didn't make any changes to her diet (like avoiding gluten), though she did continue taking folic acid. She became pregnant again almost immediately, and her second child was born the following January.

Other intriguing case reports of celiac-related folate deficiency and infertility have appeared in medical journals. For example, a twenty-nine-year-old woman who had been trying to conceive for nine years started taking folic acid to correct a type of anemia caused by too little folate in the bloodstream. A further workup showed she had celiac disease. Although she chose not to start a gluten-free diet, she became pregnant a little more than a year later.[13] Another woman saw her doctor for secondary infertility—after having a child at age twenty-three, she had not been able to get pregnant again. Blood tests and a biopsy showed she had low levels of folate and vitamin B_{12} along with signs of celiac disease. Less than a year after starting high-dose folic acid plus a gluten-free diet she became pregnant. In a fourth case, this one not involving celiac disease, a thirty-two-year-old woman who had been trying to become pregnant for ten years was started on 5,000 mg of folic acid a day because her blood folate level was quite low. Three months later she was pregnant.[13]

By themselves, case studies like these are hypothesis generating—they offer hints of a fruitful avenue for future research, not change-your-habits results. Although there has been surprisingly little follow-up on the folic acid–fertility connection, a few other lines of research bear out these cases.

Studies Lend Support

Farmers are always on the lookout for ways to make their animals more fertile. One strategy adopted by pig farmers over the past decade or so is giving sows more folic acid. The result has been more piglets in each litter.[14] It isn't clear whether folic acid does this by causing sows to release more eggs during ovulation or by helping embryos survive.

Folic Acid and Assisted Reproduction

Scottish doctors approached the question of folic acid and fertility in a novel way. They looked for links between folic acid intake and the success of IVF, which, in their clinic, usually involved the transfer of two or more fertilized eggs. The better a woman's "folate status" (higher levels of folate in the bloodstream or in red blood cells), the higher her chances of having twins as a result of IVF. The implication from this work is that having plenty of folate on board gives embryos a survival advantage.

Intrigued by the possibility that a bounty of folic acid in the body increases the chances of having twins, a team of fertility specialists in Germany wondered whether a gene involved in the production and breakdown of folate influences how the ovaries respond to follicle-stimulating hormone (FSH). This hormone, made in the pituitary gland, stimulates ovulation. The gene they focused on is methylenetetrahydrofolate reductase (MTHFR). People who carry a common variation in this gene tend to have below-normal levels of folate. Working with a group of women preparing for in vitro fertilization, the researchers measured how their ovaries responded to high doses of FSH. Women who carried the MTHFR variation required more FSH to induce ovulation, and even with higher doses they produced two to three fewer eggs than women with the usual MTHFR gene.[15] The effect was particularly strong for women over thirty-five years of age.

Not Getting Enough

Women in their childbearing years are urged to get at least 400 mcg of folic acid a day in addition to what they get from food, even if they aren't trying to get pregnant. That's because up to half of pregnancies are unplanned. Pregnant women need 600 mcg. Pregnant or not, many women don't get the folic acid they need.

Up until the late 1990s, the average American woman got only about 250 mcg of folic acid a day. In an effort to rectify this, starting in 1998 the U.S. Food and Drug Administration has required food companies to add folic acid to most enriched bread flours, cornmeal, pasta, rice, and other grain products. (See Table 8.1.) Although that has helped boost the average intake, up to two-thirds of American women still aren't getting 400 mcg a day.[16] And there is alarming information from the

Table 8.1 **Foods Rich in Folic Acid**

Grains, breads, and other foods fortified with folic acid are, along with beans and some green leafy vegetables, some of the best sources of this nutrient.

Food	Serving	Dietary Folate Equivalents (mcg)
Fortified breakfast cereals	¾ to 1 cup	200–800
White rice, enriched, cooked	1 cup	215
Lentils, cooked	½ cup	179
Pasta, cooked	1 cup	167
Garbanzo beans, cooked	½ cup	141
Spinach, cooked	½ cup	131
Asparagus, cooked	½ cup (about 6 spears)	121
Orange juice, from concentrate	6 ounces	110
Pita bread	1 piece	99
Lima beans, cooked	½ cup	78
Wheat bread	2 slices	28

Source: U.S. Department of Agriculture National Nutrient Database for Standard Reference, Release 19 (2006). (The USDA offers a free list with the folate content of hundreds of foods: www.ars.usda.gov/Services/docs .htm?docid=9673.)

Centers for Disease Control and Prevention that blood levels of folate have actually been declining in recent years, especially in women of childbearing age.[17] Low-carb diets may be to blame.

If you are having trouble getting pregnant, consider 400 mcg of folic acid taken as part of a balanced multivitamin-multimineral supplement—plus a healthful diet, of course—as a key aid. Seemingly unrelated lines of research, from studies of celiac sprue to those of gene variants, suggest that getting more folic acid can improve your chances of starting or growing a family.

▶Iron

Iron gets plenty of credit for its work inside red blood cells. There, tucked inside a protein called hemoglobin, it helps carry oxygen from the lungs to the rest of the body. But this common mineral has another equally important role in every cell in the body, from eggs and sperm to brain and heart cells. It's a tiny task: moving electrons from a high-energy molecule to a lower-energy one. Yet it is an indispensable job that allows the body to turn sugar and other fuels into adenosine triphosphate, or ATP, the energy currency of life. Iron also plays an important role in the synthesis of DNA.

Iron-poor blood is the most common nutritional deficiency in the world. It afflicts half of the earth's inhabitants, most of whom are in developing countries. Severe iron deficiency causes anemia, stunts growth, clouds the mind, causes disabling fatigue, and contributes to the deaths of thousands of women during childbirth. In the United States, iron deficiencies severe enough to cause problems like these aren't common. Mild deficiencies are, though. Up to one in seven women have below-normal levels of iron.[18] The most common cause is monthly blood loss from menstruation that isn't offset by enough iron in the diet.

A mild iron deficiency that doesn't cause anemia (too few red blood cells in circulation) isn't generally regarded as a problem. But while it may not obviously affect health, findings from the Nurses' Health Study and elsewhere suggest it may derail ovulation and make it difficult for an embryo to thrive.

Extra Iron Improves Fertility

Spurred on by hints that iron may affect fertility, we tested whether intake of this mineral influenced ovulatory infertility among women in the Nurses' Health Study.[11] It did, but in an intriguing way: the source of the iron seemed to make a difference.

As stated earlier, women who regularly took an iron supplement or a multivitamin-multimineral with extra iron (nonheme iron) were 40 percent less likely to have had trouble getting pregnant than women who didn't take iron. The benefit came with daily doses in the 40 to 80 mg range. Women who got most of their iron from meat (heme iron) weren't protected at all against ovulatory infertility, and there was a hint that high intake of iron from meat increased the chances of developing such infertility. Nonheme iron from fruits, vegetables, beans, and supplements, on the other hand, improved the chances of getting pregnant.

A connection between iron and ovulatory infertility isn't far-fetched. Human eggs (oocytes) and the granulosa cells that surround them before ovulation sport receptors for transferrin, a protein that ferries iron through the bloodstream. These receptors let oocytes grab iron from the bloodstream and store it for future use. Granulosa cells can even make their own transferrin and export it to oocytes. These are signs that the egg, and probably the embryo, need iron for the flurry of DNA and protein synthesis that happens after fertilization as well as for providing the energy to power it.

Heme and Nonheme Iron

Iron is found in every cell in the body. It exists in two forms—heme and nonheme. Heme refers to a cagelike chemical ring that holds iron in the center of a large protein. It is the centerpiece of hemoglobin, a protein in red blood cells that ferries oxygen from the lungs to cells in every part of the body. Heme, and thus iron, is also part of myoglobin, the protein that holds oxygen within the cells, especially heart and skeletal muscle cells. Much of the iron in meat is in the heme form. Nonheme iron is not bound in a cagelike ring. It is found in fruits, vegetables, grains, eggs, milk, and meat. (See Figure 8.1.)

There's another difference between the two. The body doesn't regulate the absorption of heme iron from meat as carefully as it controls

Figure 8.1 **Forms of Iron**

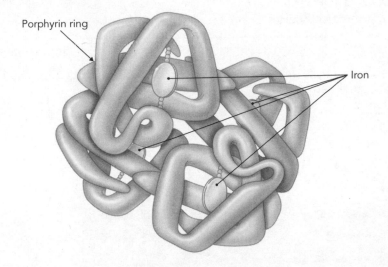

Porphyrin ring

Iron

Hemoglobin molecule

Iron is found in two forms in food and in the body. Nonheme iron is plain old iron, usually found by itself. Heme iron refers to iron embedded in a complex cagelike molecule known as a porphyrin ring that is composed of carbon, hydrogen, oxygen, and nitrogen. Heme iron is abundant in hemoglobin, the protein that carries oxygen through the bloodstream, and myoglobin, the protein in muscle and other tissues that grabs oxygen from hemoglobin.

the absorption of nonheme iron from grains, fruits, vegetables, and supplements. If your iron storehouse is well stocked, nonheme iron from plants and supplements passes out of your body in the stool. The iron in meat, though, slides under this mineral radar and adds to your stockpile, even if your body already has plenty of iron. This could be a problem if, as some research has shown, excess iron acts as a powerful generator of cell-damaging free radicals. Too much stored iron has also been linked with the development of type 2 diabetes. Good sources of nonheme iron are listed in Table 8.2.

Get an Early Start

Many women start taking a multivitamin with extra folic acid and iron once they learn they are pregnant. That's often too late. During the

Table 8.2 **Foods Rich in Nonheme Iron**

Iron is found in a multitude of foods. Fortified cereals, nuts, beans, and dried fruits are some excellent sources.

Food	Serving Size	Iron Content (mg)
Fortified breakfast cereal	1 cup	4.5–18 (check Nutrition Facts label)
Pumpkin seeds	1 ounce	4.3
Soybean nuts	½ cup	4.0
Bran	½ cup	3.5
Blackstrap molasses	1 tablespoon	3.5
Spinach, boiled	½ cup	3.2
Red kidney beans, cooked	½ cup	2.6
Lima beans, cooked	½ cup	2.5
Cashews, dry roasted	1 ounce	1.7
Enriched rice, cooked	½ cup	1.2
Raisins, seedless	⅓ cup	1.1
Prunes, dried	5 prunes	1.1
Acorn squash, baked	½ cup	1.0
Whole wheat bread	1 slice	0.9
Egg yolk	1 large yolk	0.7
White bread, made with enriched flour	1 slice	0.7
Peanut butter, chunky	2 tablespoons	0.6
Apricots, dried	3 apricots	0.6
Cod, broiled	3 ounces	0.4

Source: U.S. Department of Agriculture National Nutrient Database for Standard Reference, Release 19 (2006). (The USDA offers a free list detailing the iron content of hundreds of foods: www.ars.usda.gov/Services/docs .htm?docid=9673.)

first two to four weeks of pregnancy—a time when many women don't know they are pregnant—the embryo passes through crucial stages of development that depend on having plenty of readily available folic acid and other nutrients. New analyses show that early use of a prenatal multivitamin containing folic acid helps prevent cleft palate and other congenital birth defects, not just neural tube defects.[19,20] Being well supplied with vitamins and minerals before conception gives the fragile embryo a much-needed head start.

The findings from the Nurses' Health Study and other lines of research go a step further. They make the case that taking a prenatal vitamin while *trying* to get pregnant does double duty—it improves the odds of getting pregnant and paves the way for healthy development of a new baby.

Look for a prenatal vitamin that contains at least 400 mcg of folic acid and at least 40 mg of iron. At the same time, choose foods rich in folic acid and nonheme iron, the kind found in fruits, vegetables, beans, and nuts. Heme iron, from beef, pork, chicken, and other meats, seems to do little for fertility and may actually work against it.

▶Vitamins, Minerals, and the Y Chromosome

A daily multivitamin may improve a man's fertility as much as a woman's. Vitamins and minerals help boost the number and quality of sperm cells, two key contributors to successful conception.

It only makes sense that sperm production depends on an ample supply of micronutrients. Creating a thousand new sperm cells a second means churning out miles of DNA, a process that depends on folate, iron, zinc, and other micronutrients. The Sertoli cells in the testicles, which nurture developing sperm cells through the stages of production and maturation, have an extra need for vitamin A. Vitamin E helps immature sperm cells develop and plays a role in the secretion of prostate proteins.

The status of research on nutrition and fertility in men is even more abysmal than that in women. This makes for even more unknowns. A few rays of light are beginning to pierce the fog.

Celiac disease (discussed earlier in this chapter) affects fertility in men as much as it does in women. It does this in part by throwing off hormone levels—men with celiac disease tend to have low testosterone and high FSH. Even when the disease is under control with a gluten-free diet and hormone levels are near normal, ongoing deficiencies in folic acid, iron, and other nutrients can interfere with sperm production or maturation.

Men with certain mutations in genes that control folate metabolism have lower levels of folate in their blood than men with normal copies of these genes. Two small studies show that they are also more likely to have trouble fathering a child.[21,22] Supplementation with folic acid corrects the low folate level and may improve fertility.

Dutch researchers tested that idea by asking more than two hundred men to take unmarked pills containing either 5,000 mcg of folic acid, 66 mg of zinc, both, or a placebo for twenty-six weeks. The combination of folic acid and zinc nearly doubled the sperm count in men seeing a doctor for infertility and also increased the sperm count in fertile men, though to a lesser degree.[23]

Taking a daily multivitamin-multimineral along with your partner is a good idea. On a personal level, it's an outward show of solidarity and support. Doing it together helps you *both* remember and stick with the daily supplement. And it may boost the production of vigorous sperm cells, which can only add to your partner's efforts to improve ovulation and conception.

From a nutritional standpoint, men may benefit from a multivitamin-multimineral supplement even more than women because they tend to lag behind in eating fruits and vegetables, the key sources of vitamins and minerals. More than 80 percent of men don't get the recommended five fruits and vegetables a day,[24] opening the door to vitamin and mineral shortages that a supplement can correct.

But don't take your partner's prenatal vitamin. Men don't need as much iron as women do, and they definitely don't need as much as found in most prenatal pills. A standard multivitamin-multimineral will do. It also offers extra folic acid, zinc, and other vitamins and minerals that may improve sperm production and quality.

Chapter 9
· · · · · · · ·

Drink (Water) to Your Health

KEY STRATEGY

Drink coffee or tea in moderation. Cut back on sugared sodas. Alcohol? There's no simple answer.

The key message about diet from the Nurses' Health Study is clear: what you eat can affect your chances of getting pregnant. How about what you drink? Can that make a difference, too?

It can. Staying hydrated is important for fertility and general good health. As we described in Chapter 7, drinking a glass of whole milk every day can improve ovulatory function and help stave off infertility. The two beverages most women want to know about—coffee and alcohol—also influence fertility, although not quite as much as the headlines and "commonsense advice" would have you believe.

One minor theme we've sounded in the preceding chapters is how little research has been done on connections between nutrition and fertility. Water and other beverages get barely a footnote. Coffee and alcohol are the exceptions. Dozens of studies have looked at their effects on fertility and pregnancy. Unfortunately, the often contradictory results have created more confusion than solution about these popular beverages.

In this chapter we make the case for coffee and tea that you can take them—in moderation—or leave them. Soft drinks, on the other hand, are better left unopened. The picture for alcohol is still hazy. We didn't see any harmful effects of alcohol on fertility in the Nurses' Health Study, which offers reassurance for women who enjoy a drink now and then. But others may feel better abstaining from alcohol.

▶Staying Hydrated

Face cream, hand lotion, lip balm—many women consider these essentials for keeping their skin moist and soft. Few give much thought to the body's true moisturizers: the fluids they drink.

More than half of your body weight is a salty liquid that resembles the seawater that first nourished life. This liquid gives cells their shape and solidity. It bathes, cushions, and lubricates tissues and organs. It forms the supply routes for nutrients, the disposal system for wastes, and a watery communication system for hormones and other signaling molecules. Bodily fluids are so precious that your skin, nasal passages, kidneys, and a number of hormones work together to keep their amount and chemical composition as stable and unchanging as possible.

You play a role as well. You need to take in enough fluid each day to replenish what's lost when you exhale, sweat, or urinate. How much you need depends on what you eat, how active you are, and the temperature and humidity. As a general rule, you need a milliliter of water for every calorie you burn. If you take in two thousand calories a day, you need at least two thousand milliliters of fluid, or about sixty-four ounces—more if you are very active or the temperature is high. Some of that liquid can come from food. Fruits, vegetables, soups, and salads are flavorful sources of water. The rest must come from beverages. Some beverages are better than others. By better we mean they give you what you need—water—without adding calories or other things that might derail health or fertility.

Every four years the dedicated volunteers in the Nurses' Health Study offer a snapshot of their daily beverage consumption. One in six of the participants in the fertility study are confirmed water drinkers, downing six or more glasses a day. Others love coffee, tea, or soda. Many drink alcohol, usually wine, several times a week. This variety gave us the ability to look for connections between fertility and intake of caffeine or alcohol, two very controversial substances in pregnancy and fertility research. We also searched for links between individual beverages such as coffee, tea, soda, and wine.

The results, in a nutshell, were a bit surprising.[1] We found that moderate alcohol consumption (up to a drink or two a day) had little effect on overall fertility or problems with ovulation. The same was true for coffee and tea in moderation (several cups a day). Caffeine—from caffeinated soft drinks, not coffee or tea—diminished fertility in general, but not ovulatory fertility. And sugared sodas appeared to promote ovulatory infertility.

For all of the other elements of the Fertility Diet, our findings from the Nurses' Health Study represent one of the very few pieces of a puzzle on diet and fertility that we hope will be solved as others explore more fully the connections between the two. That isn't the case for caffeine and alcohol. Dozens of previous studies have looked at their impact on fertility and pregnancy, with no clear resolution in sight. Our findings are just one piece of this vast puzzle. We believe they offer reassurance that moderate intake of caffeine and alcohol are not deterrents to fertility.

▶Caffeine

Caffeine is the world's most popular mind-altering drug. It's the reason people the world over gulp coffee, tea, colas, cocoa, yerba maté, and other plant-based drinks. Most do it for the gentle pick-me-up that caffeine offers. Some say that caffeine helps them stay alert or concentrate better. Others drink coffee, tea, soda, or other caffeinated beverages because they like the way they taste. Whatever the reason, nearly 90 percent of American adults report using caffeine in one form or another every day.

Of course, caffeine doesn't affect just the mind. It revs up the central nervous system, increases the heart rate, and relaxes smooth muscles, like those lining blood vessels. These changes are usually subtle. Get too much caffeine, though, and you'll feel your heart race and get the jitters. The reverse of these side effects accounts for the caffeine withdrawal that some people experience when they don't get their morning jolt. This appears in the form of a nasty headache, drowsiness, unhappiness, irritability, or difficulty concentrating.

When you drink coffee, tea, or another caffeinated beverage, its caffeine quickly courses through your body. It enters the ovary, uterus, and fallopian tubes, along with just about every other tissue. Caffeine has been found in newly fertilized eggs and embryos. It crosses the placenta, giving developing babies their own tiny buzz, as shown by an increase in fetal heart rate and changes in the baby's movement patterns.

Caffeine's reputation as being hazardous during pregnancy comes from a shocking study done in 1980. FDA researchers force-fed pregnant rats with the caffeine equivalent of two hundred cups of coffee a day. The study found that one of every five baby rats born to these mothers had permanent birth defects—mainly missing or incomplete toes.[2] That prompted the FDA to warn pregnant women to avoid caffeine or cut back on it. When the same researchers repeated the study two years later, this time putting caffeine in the rats' water supply and letting them drink at will, there was no increase in birth defects.[3] Yet the FDA didn't change its advice.

Since then, researchers have tried mightily to pin down caffeine's impact on fertility and pregnancy. The steady drip, drip, drip of results hasn't yielded a single firm conclusion. Some studies show that caffeine in moderation (which usually means under 300 mg a day, the equivalent of two to three regular cups of coffee) has no effect on fertility, successful pregnancy, or fetal development. Others suggest that it slightly delays pregnancy and poses a small risk to the developing child. Imbibing a lot of caffeine every day may increase the risks of miscarriage, preterm delivery, and low birth weight, but again there is no rock-solid proof of this.

We investigated the connection between caffeine and fertility in the Nurses' Health Study. Caffeine didn't appear to affect ovulation. Women in the high-caffeine group, who got more than 400 mg of caffeine a day (the equivalent of four cups of coffee), were no more likely to have had problems with ovulatory infertility than women who got barely any caffeine. But when we looked at all causes of infertility, women in the high-caffeine group were about 20 percent more likely to have had trouble getting pregnant. It is possible that too much caffeine makes the fallopian tubes less able to contract and relax, which could slow the transit of a fertilized egg from the tube to the uterus. If the egg arrives too late, the endometrium might no longer be receptive to its implantation. Caffeine could also make the endometrium less hospitable to a fertilized egg.[4]

A similar connection has been seen before, in a study that compared caffeine intake among more than one thousand women who attended an infertility clinic and another four thousand matched for age and other characteristics who had babies at a nearby hospital. High intake of caffeine was linked with infertility due to tubal problems or endometriosis but was not associated with ovulatory infertility.[5]

To get at whether caffeine itself or a particular caffeinated beverage was the culprit, we ran the numbers separately for each caffeinated beverage. It turned out that only caffeinated soft drinks were related to infertility. Once we removed them from the picture using statistical techniques, caffeine was no longer related to infertility of any kind.

Why Such Confusion?

With all of the research on caffeine and reproduction, why is there no consensus about its effects? Timing may have an effect. How a woman metabolizes caffeine changes throughout her menstrual cycle. There's a marked slowdown during the luteal phase, which begins the day after ovulation, that may lead to higher levels of caffeine in the body during the period of fertilization, implantation, and early embryonic development.[6] Another problem may well be genetic—some women break down caffeine faster than others and so may be less prone to any possible negative effects.

It's possible that the contradictory results may stem more from methodology than from biology. How a study is conducted can affect its results. In studies of nutrition and health problems, whether diet is measured before the outcome (like infertility or cancer) or after can make a big difference. Assessing diet after the fact introduces the very real possibility that people will recall their diets through the lens of their health problem, possibly looking for a way to blame it on something. Measuring it beforehand avoids this bias.

Let's take a look at the fourteen studies that had explored a connection between coffee or caffeine intake and fertility before we take a look in the Nurses' Health Study. Eight of them indicated that caffeine or coffee diminished fertility; in six of these, diet information was collected from the participants after they had been diagnosed with infertility. Contrast this with the findings of the five studies in which dietary data were collected before women started trying to get pregnant: two suggested that coffee and caffeine may hamper fertility, two found no connection between coffee or caffeine and fertility, and one suggested that consuming three to seven cups of coffee a day actually improved fertility! Add our results to the "assess diet beforehand" group, and there is just as much evidence that coffee or caffeine has no effect on fertility as there is that it may impair it.

Calming the Caffeine Jitters

On the surface, caffeine consumption in the Nurses' Health Study looked as though it held back fertility. Once caffeinated soft drinks were taken out of the picture, though, the connection between caffeine and fertility melted away. This should be reassuring to coffee and tea drinkers.

Reassurance doesn't mean carte blanche to guzzle. If these brews are beverages you savor, you need not deny yourself the pleasure of their company. Just don't go overboard—we didn't see any effects on fertility at moderate levels of caffeine intake, which is the equivalent of three to four cups of coffee a day. If you prefer to err on the side of caution, try decaffeinated coffee or tea, cut back on your intake, or give them up altogether if it will make you feel more secure. If you rely on caffeinated and sugared sodas, though, a temporary switch to a sugar-free soda or another beverage altogether while you are trying to get pregnant might make sense.

▶Coffee

A cup of coffee delivers mostly water. Taken black without sugar, it is nearly calorie free. It is brimming with antioxidants and other biologically active substances, including caffeine. Several long-term studies have shown that coffee drinkers are less likely to develop type 2 diabetes, gallstones and kidney stones, and possibly colon cancer. The main downsides of coffee drinking are caffeine addiction and the fats and calories that come with the sugar, cream, whipped cream, caramel, and other toppings and flavoring now put in and on coffee.

Almost half of the women in the Nurses' Health Study say they drink coffee every day. In the fertility study, the coffee drinkers weren't any more or less likely to have had trouble getting pregnant than women who didn't drink coffee. Ovulation-related infertility was similar across the spectrum of coffee drinking, as was infertility due to other causes, such as endometriosis or tubal problems. That held for caffeinated and decaffeinated coffee, at least up to two or three cups a day. Few of the women in the study drank more than that, so we can't say much about the effects on fertility of pot-a-day coffee habits.

These results don't solve the "Should I quit coffee or not?" dilemma that women face when they are trying to get pregnant. But they do add to the rather substantial body of evidence that a cup or two of coffee a day has no effect on fertility.

What about coffee during pregnancy? Most major studies have found no connection between moderate coffee drinking and preterm delivery, birth defects, or delivering a baby with a low birth weight. Most studies investigating a possible link between caffeine and mis-

CAFFEINE VARIATIONS

Estimating your caffeine intake can be tricky. Few soft drinks print their caffeine content on the label, and the caffeine content of coffee varies wildly. Brewed at home, the average eight-ounce cup of coffee contains between 80 and 120 mg of coffee. Yet many people drink coffee by the sixteen-ounce mug.

What's in restaurant coffee is anyone's guess. A University of Florida team highlighted the variation by analyzing the caffeine in coffees brewed by different companies. A sixteen-ounce cup of Starbucks Breakfast Blend bought from the same store on six consecutive days ranged from a whopping 564 mg of caffeine to a "low" of 259 mg. Among other brewed coffees, a sixteen-ounce Dunkin' Donuts regular contained 143 mg.[7] It's enough to make you switch to tea.

carriage show a connection between the two. However, problems with study design make it impossible to know if this is a true cause-and-effect relationship.

Coffee is the most important source of caffeine for the majority of Americans. So our recommendation about safe amounts for fertility follow what we said earlier for caffeine—be moderate. Our findings from the Nurses' Health Study indicate that having two or three cups of coffee a day has no effect on fertility. If you don't like to take chances and can give up the bean, switch to decaf or give up coffee altogether. The same advice holds for when you get pregnant.

▶Tea for Two?

After water, tea is the second-most commonly imbibed beverage in the world. Numerous health benefits have been ascribed to tea drinking. Like coffee, it almost certainly helps prevent kidney stones and gallstones. There is also some evidence that drinking tea offers protection against heart disease, stroke, and some cancers, especially stomach cancer, but this is still in flux.

Its international popularity aside, tea trails coffee in the United States and in the Nurses' Health Study. Still, almost one-quarter of the participants drink a cup or two of tea every day. Like coffee, tea appears to have no effect on fertility. Women who said they drank it at least twice a day were no more likely to have had problems with infertility than women who didn't drink tea at all.

Research over the years has drawn an uncertain line between tea drinking and fertility. In some studies tea had no effect on pregnancy rates. In others it was linked with a decrease in fertility. One report, from a large California health maintenance organization, went the other direction, showing that drinking a cup of tea a day doubled the odds of conception.[8]

If English breakfast tea is what gets you started in the morning, Earl Grey eases your afternoons, or Constant Comment fires you up for a chat, drink with gusto and rest easy that your fertility isn't slipping away. You probably don't want to have six cups to be "in touch with the immortals," as poet Lu Tong wrote more than twelve hundred years ago, but several cups a day—moderate consumption—should be fine. If you prefer to be extra cautious and minimize even the remote possibility that tea might curb your fertility, then give it up.

▶Soda

While coffee, tea, and alcohol don't seem to affect fertility, sodas sure do. Among women in the Nurses' Health Study, those who drank two or more caffeinated sodas a day were 50 percent more likely to have experienced ovulatory infertility than women who drank these less than once a week. We suspected that something other than caffeine was driving this connection for two reasons: these were the only caffeinated beverages that affected fertility, and caffeinated sodas usually have much less caffeine than coffee. So we looked at noncaffeinated sodas to see if there was any connection with their consumption. And we saw the same interference with fertility. Finally, when we statistically accounted for caffeine in soda (in a sense removing it from playing a role in soda's reproductive effects), the link between drinking soda and infertility actually became stronger.

Although this work doesn't tell us what it is about sodas that affects fertility, it indicates that it almost surely isn't caffeine.

The sugar and caloric punch of regular soft drinks could be a contributor. On average, a twelve-ounce soda delivers 150 to 200 calories, thanks to the nine to eleven teaspoons of rapidly digested sugar it contains. These empty calories make blood sugar and insulin levels spike immediately, and over the long term they can contribute to weight gain. Both the blood sugar roller coaster and the extra pounds can get in the way of becoming pregnant.

If you prefer to slake your thirst with soft drinks, try switching to diet soda while trying to get pregnant. You can also get the fizz without the sugar buzz by mixing seltzer water with a splash of lemon, lime, orange, grape, or grapefruit juice. Such homemade spritzers offer a tasty, low-calorie thirst quencher that will avoid most of the problems with soft drinks.

▶Alcohol

Heavy drinking is indisputably harmful—for general health, mental health, relationships, and reproduction. It can halt menstrual periods, stop ovulation, throw off the hormone cycles needed for conception and the implantation of a fertilized egg, end a pregnancy with miscarriage, and trigger early menopause. Alcohol abuse can endanger a new life from the moment of conception until after birth.

Whether *moderate* drinking—say, a glass a day (see Figure 9.1)—has similar effects is a seemingly innocent and scientific question that conceals a maelstrom of controversy. Dozens of studies have looked at the impact of moderate drinking on fertility and fetal development. The results are all over the map. Some show that women who are moderate drinkers take longer to get pregnant than nondrinkers.[9] In a study conducted among women undergoing IVF, those who drank alcohol in the month before the IVF cycle produced fewer eggs and had lower pregnancy rates. In another study, moderate drinking didn't affect fertility among women under age thirty but did get in the way of pregnancy for older women.[10] Other studies show the opposite. In a Danish study, women who were moderate drinkers averaging a drink a day got pregnant *faster* than teetotalers.[11] In another study, women who drank wine got pregnant faster than nondrinkers or those who drank beer or spirits.[12] It's no wonder that some experts warn that even a single drink before or during pregnancy can cause harm while others say the occasional drink is fine.

Figure 9.1 **What Is "a Drink"?**

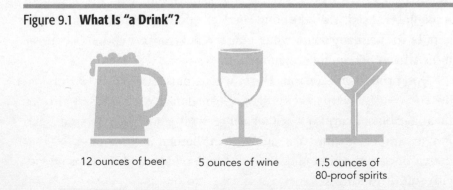

12 ounces of beer   5 ounces of wine   1.5 ounces of
                                                     80-proof spirits

Results from the Nurses' Health Study provide another piece of the puzzle, but only for very moderate drinking, up to one drink a day. When we divided the women into five groups based on their daily alcohol intake, the heaviest drinkers took in thirteen grams of alcohol a day, or just under a drink a day. This would classify them as what the Centers for Disease Control and Prevention would call light to moderate drinkers.

Infertility due to problems with ovulation was no more common among nurses who had a drink a day than it was among those who didn't drink alcohol at all. The same was true for infertility due to endometriosis, blocked fallopian tubes, and other causes. It didn't matter what kind of alcoholic beverages the women preferred. A daily glass of wine, beer, or spirits didn't seem to help or hinder getting pregnant.

How do these results fit in with earlier work? Of fifteen studies of a possible connection between alcohol intake and fertility, eight reported a potentially harmful effect. Four of the eight asked women about their alcohol consumption after they had been diagnosed with infertility. As mentioned earlier, this "look-back" approach can introduce a subtle but very real bias as women try to find reasons for their difficulty conceiving. The tendency is to exaggerate things that might have been harmful. Among the six studies that collected information on alcohol consumption before the participants started trying to get pregnant (as we did), four found that alcohol might impair fertility and two found no connection between alcohol and fertility. Adding our results to these findings doesn't do much to resolve the issue.

Beyond Conception

Conception is just the first step of a nine-month journey for a woman and her baby. Heavy drinking can derail pregnancy with a miscarriage or a stillbirth. It can also harm a fetus in several ways. Alcohol passes quickly through the placenta. An unborn baby breaks down alcohol much more slowly than its mother, so the alcohol level in its blood can reach high levels even when the mother's is still OK. This can lead to fetal alcohol syndrome, a condition that causes lifelong physical and mental disabilities. Heavy drinking can also lead to more subtle problems with thinking skills and behavior. No one really knows if moderate, responsible drinking has similar effects on pregnancy and the development of a new life.

Timing is one issue. It is possible, though not proven, that alcohol prevents nerves from making essential connections in the growing brain at certain critical moments of fetal development but has little or no effect at other times. A mother's metabolism is another unknown. Women whose bodies break down alcohol quickly may be able to drink safely throughout pregnancy, while those who metabolize it more slowly may need to abstain.[13] But there isn't an easy way to know what stage of brain development your baby is in or how your body handles alcohol, or to tell precisely when you became pregnant.

Given the uncertainties about alcohol and reproduction, the safest course of action is to temporarily forgo wine, beer, or other alcoholic beverages while you are trying to get pregnant. Alcohol certainly doesn't *promote* fertility, so you aren't missing anything vital by giving it up. To be sure, a glass of wine can help set a romantic mood or ease the stress that sometimes accompanies infertility. But there are alternatives, like a massage for mood or exercise for stress. To minimize any possible hazards of alcohol for a fertilized egg or new fetus, when trying to conceive, treat your body as if you were pregnant, since you could be pregnant at any time.

But if you do have a drink, enjoy it with your head held high. There is no evidence that having a drink every now and then when trying to get pregnant will stop your quest in its tracks. If that was the case, a nightly glass of wine would have been discovered eons ago as an easy form of birth control.

▶Men Drink, Too

Caffeine and alcohol affect men much as they do women. Both have even been implicated in male reproduction. Early studies showing that caffeine improved the swimming ability of sperm led to its use for a while in the fluid used to bathe sperm during in vitro fertilization. Caffeine's effect on sperm development or maturation in the testicles, though, remains largely a mystery. If caffeine affects a man's fertility, and that's a big *if,* the effect is small.

Alcohol at levels that harm the liver and other organs can definitely reduce fertility in men. Alcohol abuse can lower testosterone levels, shrink the testicles, make it difficult to get or sustain an erection, and slow sperm production.[14] The effect of *moderate* drinking on fertility, though, is as uncertain in men as it is in women. Some work suggests it is a hazard. A Danish study that tracked conception and early miscarriage by testing participants' urine samples for pregnancy hormones found more miscarriages among women whose partners had two or more drinks a day in the month before conception.[15] California researchers showed that among couples undergoing in vitro fertilization, those in which the male partner routinely drank alcohol were less likely to have a successful pregnancy than those in which the man didn't drink alcohol.[16] Other studies found no effects of moderate drinking among men on the number, quality, or swimming ability of sperm, conception rates, or miscarriage.

Limiting coffee and alcohol may improve a man's fertility. Then again, it may not. So we offer the same advice to men as we do to women: if pregnancy is your goal, the most prudent course of action is to keep your intake of caffeine and alcohol in the moderate range. If, like your partner, you want to avoid even the semblance of risk, give them up altogether.

Chapter 10

The 7½ Percent Solution

KEY STRATEGY

Aim for a body weight in the "fertility zone." Even small changes in that direction can make a big difference.

In the solar system of the body, weight is the sun—the keeper of stored energy that influences the orbits of the planets of health. Reproduction, the Venus of this system, is exquisitely affected by the gravitational pull of weight. Weighing too much or too little can interrupt normal menstrual cycles, throw off ovulation, or stop it altogether. Excess weight lowers the odds that in vitro fertilization or other assisted reproductive technologies will succeed. It increases the chances of miscarriage, puts a mother at risk during pregnancy of developing high blood pressure (preeclampsia) or diabetes, and elevates her chances of needing a Cesarean section.[1] The dangers of being overweight or underweight extend to a woman's baby as well, as described in "Starting Early."

Weight isn't an issue just for women or limited to reproduction. Budding research indicates that overweight men aren't as fertile as their healthy-weight counterparts, with excess weight lowering sperm production. Weight directly and indirectly influences many other aspects of health. As shown in Figure 10.1, more than fifty different medical conditions have been linked with excess weight, from breathing problems (asthma) to circulatory disorders (heart attack, high blood pressure, heart failure), muscle and joint problems (arthritis), and digestive

Figure 10.1 **Obesity's Long Reach**

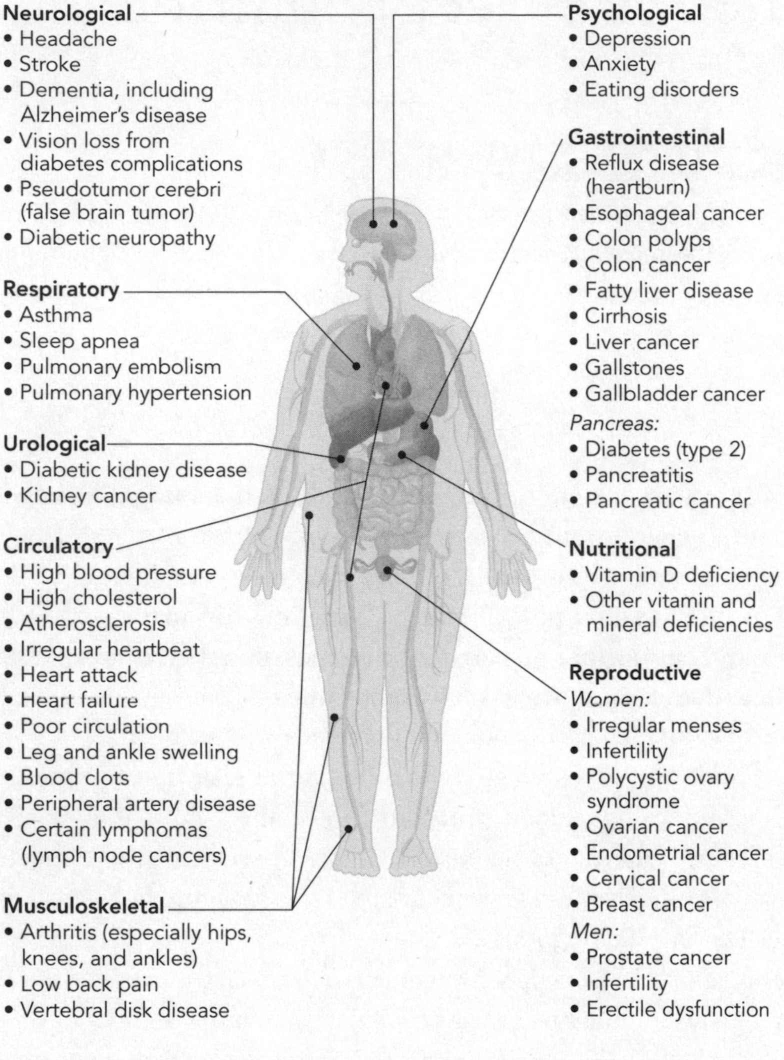

Neurological
- Headache
- Stroke
- Dementia, including
  Alzheimer's disease
- Vision loss from
  diabetes complications
- Pseudotumor cerebri
  (false brain tumor)
- Diabetic neuropathy

Respiratory
- Asthma
- Sleep apnea
- Pulmonary embolism
- Pulmonary hypertension

Urological
- Diabetic kidney disease
- Kidney cancer

Circulatory
- High blood pressure
- High cholesterol
- Atherosclerosis
- Irregular heartbeat
- Heart attack
- Heart failure
- Poor circulation
- Leg and ankle swelling
- Blood clots
- Peripheral artery disease
- Certain lymphomas
  (lymph node cancers)

Musculoskeletal
- Arthritis (especially hips,
  knees, and ankles)
- Low back pain
- Vertebral disk disease

Psychological
- Depression
- Anxiety
- Eating disorders

Gastrointestinal
- Reflux disease
  (heartburn)
- Esophageal cancer
- Colon polyps
- Colon cancer
- Fatty liver disease
- Cirrhosis
- Liver cancer
- Gallstones
- Gallbladder cancer

Pancreas:
- Diabetes (type 2)
- Pancreatitis
- Pancreatic cancer

Nutritional
- Vitamin D deficiency
- Other vitamin and
  mineral deficiencies

Reproductive
Women:
- Irregular menses
- Infertility
- Polycystic ovary
  syndrome
- Ovarian cancer
- Endometrial cancer
- Cervical cancer
- Breast cancer

Men:
- Prostate cancer
- Infertility
- Erectile dysfunction

Obesity, defined as having a BMI of 30 or greater, affects nearly every system in the body. It increases the chances of developing scores of diseases, from stroke and Alzheimer's disease to poor circulation in the feet.

ailments (colon cancer, gastroesophageal reflux disease). Being overweight can interfere with sleep, make it difficult to keep up physically with children or friends, and shorten life.

▶Roots of the Problem

Body weight is an imprecise blend of nature and nurture. The effects and interactions of these two determine why some people can eat anything they want—ice cream, pizza, pasta, you name it—and never gain weight while others pack on the pounds no matter how carefully they seem to eat.

Genes are the nature part. So far, scientists have discovered more than four hundred genes that may contribute to the development of overweight or obesity. They affect appetite; metabolism; food cravings; satiety (the sense of fullness after eating); where the body stores fat; the production of hormones such as insulin, insulin-like growth factor, leptin, and their receptors; and even the tendency to use eating as a way to cope with stress. In most people, genes contribute only a bit to weight and weight gain. In others, they are 80 percent responsible for weight. Having a rough idea of how large a role genes play in your weight may be helpful in terms of shedding pounds.

For most people, nurture—the environment—has the biggest impact on weight. The effect starts early, sometimes even before birth. Babies of women who smoke during pregnancy, or who have diabetes, or who

HOW MUCH OF YOUR WEIGHT DEPENDS ON YOUR GENES?

Your weight may be largely the product of your genes if:

- You have been overweight for much of your life.
- One or both of your parents or several other blood relatives are or have been substantially overweight.
- Losing weight is almost impossible even when you *faithfully* stick to a low-calorie diet and increase your physical activity.

Just because genes may play a relatively large role in determining your weight doesn't mean you are incapable of controlling your weight. It does mean you need extra help from a nutritionist, a doctor, family members, and friends to do it.

STARTING EARLY

You can probably pinpoint the most important few months of your life—your first love, a period of athletic or scholastic achievement, a huge project at work, planning a wedding. Developmentally speaking, the most important few months of your life happened before you were born. That's when every system in your body was formed and programmed for the future.

In the late 1980s, David Barker, a British physician, wondered if the "decisions" made by a developing child could affect his or her health as an adult. This thought came from his observation that low-weight babies tend to grow into adults who are prone to high blood pressure and heart disease. That idea, explored and tested by hundreds of researchers since, has blossomed into what's known as the fetal origins hypothesis.

It goes like this: a fetus faced with poor nutrition—either too little food or poor quality food—chooses to use it in ways that will maximize its early survival. One way this happens is that the fetus's tissues become somewhat resistant to insulin, the hormone needed to usher blood sugar into muscle and other cells. Blood sugar levels remain high, making it easier for brain cells (which don't need insulin to sponge up blood sugar) to get the energy they need. The nutritional environment in the uterus also activates genes that make it easier for the fetus to store body fat later in life. These adaptations make perfect sense if the environment into which the child is born is one where food is sometimes scarce. But when the environment is one of calorie-laden fast food and nearly nonstop eating, these traits can lead to trouble, especially diabetes, high blood pressure, and becoming overweight.

are overweight are more likely to become overweight during childhood or later in life. During infancy, breast-feeding offers some protection against childhood obesity. During childhood, being rewarded or punished with food can lead to unhealthy eating habits, while family practices such as rarely sitting down together for dinner or habits such as drinking a lot of juice or sugary sodas can lead to excess weight. The sheer amount of food available to us at every turn—in restaurants, the mall, even gas stations—makes it difficult to *not* gain weight. But wait, there's more! As a nation we are exercising less and spending more time in front of the television or computer. And we are hurrying more, for work and for family, leading us to eat on the run, sacrifice sleep, and be stressed out, all of which can contribute to weight gain. No wonder the American environment has been called "obesogenic," meaning likely to cause someone to become fat.

What Is a Healthy Weight?

There isn't a single answer to the question "What is a healthy weight?" It varies from individual to individual because it depends on height and other factors. What may be a perfect weight for a tall person may be way too much for a shorter one or one with less muscle.

A measure called the body mass index (BMI) combines height and weight into a single number. By adjusting for the fact that taller people should weigh more than shorter people, the BMI makes it easier to compare people of different heights and come up with healthy weight guidelines. It is a good indicator of total body fat, which is related to the risk of disease and death. Although BMI tends to overestimate body fat in athletes and others who have a muscular build and under-estimate it in older individuals and those who have lost muscle mass, it is remarkably reliable for most of us.

OVERWEIGHT OR OBESE?

In plain language, being overweight means weighing more than you "should." The term actually has a more precise meaning, at least in the context of nutrition and medicine. *Overweight* refers to being modestly above what's considered a healthy weight for your frame. In terms of body mass index (BMI), you are overweight if your BMI is between 25 and 29.9. *Obese* refers to being substantially above the healthy weight range, with a BMI of 30 or higher. We'll use the term *overweight* to refer to everyone above the healthy weight range and *obese* or *obesity* only when needed.

You can calculate your BMI like this: multiply your weight in pounds by 703, divide that number by your height in inches, and then divide again by your height in inches. You can also look it up in Figure 10.2 or use one of many online calculators, such as the one posted by the National Heart, Lung, and Blood Institute at www.nhlbisupport. com/bmi.

Health and nutrition experts have been grappling with the healthy weight question for decades. Some of the earliest answers actually came from the life insurance industry. Statisticians called actuaries

Figure 10.2 **Finding Your BMI**

Height	Weight in pounds													
4'10"	91	96	100	105	110	115	119	124	129	134	138	143	167	191
4'11"	94	99	104	109	114	119	124	128	133	138	143	148	173	198
5'0"	97	102	107	112	118	123	128	133	138	143	148	153	179	204
5'1"	100	106	111	116	122	127	132	137	143	148	153	158	185	211
5'2"	104	109	115	120	126	131	136	142	147	153	158	164	191	218
5'3"	107	113	118	124	130	135	141	146	152	158	163	169	197	225
5'4"	110	116	122	128	134	140	145	151	157	163	169	174	204	232
5'5"	114	120	126	132	138	144	150	156	162	168	174	180	210	240
5'6"	118	124	130	136	142	148	155	161	167	173	179	186	216	247
5'7"	121	127	134	140	146	153	159	166	172	178	185	191	223	255
5'8"	125	131	138	144	151	158	164	171	177	184	190	197	230	262
5'9"	128	135	142	149	155	162	169	176	182	189	196	203	236	270
5'10"	132	139	146	153	160	167	174	181	188	195	202	207	243	278
5'11"	136	143	150	157	165	172	179	186	193	200	208	215	250	286
6'0"	140	147	154	162	169	177	184	191	199	206	213	221	258	294
6'1"	144	151	159	166	174	182	189	197	204	212	219	227	265	302
6'2"	148	155	163	171	179	186	194	202	210	218	225	233	272	311
6'3"	152	160	168	176	184	192	200	208	216	224	232	240	279	319
6'4"	156	164	172	180	189	197	205	213	221	230	238	246	287	328
BMI	19	20	21	22	23	24	25	26	27	28	29	30	35	40
	Healthy Weight						Overweight					Obese		

Your body mass index (BMI): Are you a healthy weight?

☐ Healthy weight, 18.5–24   ☐ Overweight, 25–29   ☐ Obese, 30+

To use this table, first weigh yourself without clothes and measure your height without shoes. Find your height in the left-hand column. Follow across until you hit the box with the weight closest to yours. Your BMI will be at the bottom of that column. For example, if you are five feet six inches tall and weigh 165 pounds, you would scan across to the 167 box and then look down to a BMI of 27.

Source: Dietary Guidelines for Americans, 2005.

compiled information on weight and height for thousands of people to see if weight was linked to health or survival (a useful bit of information for an insurance company). Beginning in the 1940s, the Metropolitan Life Insurance Company started publishing tables with "ideal" and "desirable" weights associated with the lowest death rates. Several more recent studies have taken this early work a big step further. These studies correlated the BMIs of millions of people with rates of illness and death. The range associated with the least illness and lowest rate of premature death is 18.5 to 24.9. That's why BMIs between 18.5 and 24.9 have been designated as the healthy range. A person who is five feet five inches and weighs 114 pounds would have a BMI of 19, while someone who is five feet five inches and weighs 150 pounds would have a BMI of 25. As BMI increases above 25, so does the risk of dying early, especially from heart disease, stroke, or cancer. The risks are even higher with BMIs above 30. People with BMIs of 25 to 29.9 are considered overweight and those with BMIs of 30 or higher are considered to be obese. Obesity has been parsed into mild (BMI of 30–34.9), moderate (35–39.9), and severe (40 and above). Severe obesity is roughly equivalent to being eighty pounds overweight if you are a woman or one hundred pounds overweight if you are a man.

Individuals with BMIs under 18.5 are considered underweight. Older studies showed that being too thin was linked to early death from heart disease, cancer, and other chronic conditions. But much of this work didn't take into consideration the fact that smokers tend to be leaner than nonsmokers and that many people inadvertently lose weight as a result of undiagnosed cancers and other conditions. In newer studies that accounted for smoking and undiagnosed disease, healthy nonsmokers with stable BMIs under 18.5 appeared to live long, healthy lives.

▶A Healthy Middle Matters, Too

Some people store much of their fat around the waist and chest; others store it around the hips and thighs. These two different body shapes have been dubbed apple and pear.

WHERE'S YOUR WAIST?

Measuring your waist doesn't mean checking your pants size. That's usually the *narrowest* part of your torso. Instead, it involves wrapping a flexible measuring tape around your midsection, even with the top of your hip bone. The tape will probably pass near your navel. Keep the tape parallel to the floor as it encircles your waist.

Fat that accumulates around the waist and chest, technically called abdominal adiposity, may pose more of a health problem than fat around the hips and thighs. It has been linked with high blood pressure, high cholesterol, high blood sugar, and heart disease. Belly fat, especially the visceral fat that surrounds the organs in the gut, secretes molecules that rev up inflammation throughout the body. In addition to promoting heart disease and diabetes, this burden of inflammation can also muffle ovulation.

Keeping track of your waist can be useful because many people convert muscle to abdominal fat as they age. Even though weight may remain stable, an expanding waistline can be a warning sign of trouble on the horizon. You can use your waist as a kind of low-tech biofeedback device—a waist-wise expansion of two or three inches over the years should trigger a warning that you need to reevaluate your diet and physical activity level.

The same national guidelines that mapped out worrisome levels of weight have also identified worrisome waist sizes.[2] A woman with a waist greater than thirty-five inches or a man with one larger than forty inches is at risk for heart disease, type 2 diabetes, and other chronic conditions. But don't wait to hit these limits before taking action, because most people will experience some increase in risk before reaching these measurements.

As far as we can tell, no studies have linked a woman's waistline with fertility. In women with polycystic ovary syndrome, though, waist circumference has a stronger influence on resistance to insulin—which can impinge on ovulation—than does body mass index. If that's also the case for women without polycystic ovary syndrome, then a large waist could impair ovulation.

▶ What Is a Healthy Weight for Fertility?

Pregnancy takes energy, literally and figuratively. For our hunter-gatherer ancestors, the physical demands of pregnancy would have been easier to bear when food was plentiful and likely to remain that way. But when it was scarce, pregnancy would have been doubly difficult for mother and child and maybe even for the whole family unit. This is reflected in the exquisite lines of communication between the reproductive system and energy stores. A host of hormones provide feedback between the two that help determine fertility. Weight, or BMI, is an outward sign of this communication.

This is easiest to understand with undernutrition. As fat stores dwindle, menstruation and ovulation falter. At some point, they cease altogether. This makes sense from an evolutionary point of view—the body temporarily stops putting energy into reproduction and instead uses it for gathering food, staying warm, and running the rest of the body. A famine that affected the Netherlands near the end of World War II is one of many examples of this effect. Between October 1944 and January 1945, the average intake of food fell from fifteen hundred calories a day to seven hundred. Nine months after the famine started, the birth rate plummeted dramatically.[3] As we describe in Chapter 11, you can see the effect today in women with anorexia, and sometimes in elite athletes, who stop menstruating when they become too light or too lean.

What about overnutrition? If stored energy is a good thing, then women with a lot of it should be extremely fertile. That's not the case. As weight climbs, so do levels of insulin and insulin-like growth factor-1, while sex hormone binding globulin declines. The net result of these changes is an increase in the amount of free and active testosterone and other male sex hormones in the ovaries and the bloodstream. This can dampen ovulation and can lead to delays in getting pregnant or block it altogether.

The body's storehouse for extra energy is adipose tissue, more commonly known as body fat. Long thought of as merely a passive depot, body fat is turning out to be an active and complex tissue. Like the pancreas or hypothalamus, adipose tissue generates a variety of hormones that influence appetite, activity, weight, and reproduction. Adiponectin is the most abundant protein made by fat cells. It helps stimulate fat-burning processes, makes cells more sensitive to insulin, and may enhance ovulation.[4] The more weight you gain, though, the less adiponectin your fat cells make. This drop-off can contribute to insulin resistance and interfere with ovulation. It also elevates leptin and other hormones that disrupt ovulation. Extra body fat boosts levels of interleukin-6 and other cell-signaling molecules that interfere with the ability of a fertilized egg to implant itself in the lining of the uterus. The main hormones secreted by fat cells and their effects on reproduction are listed in Table 10.1.

Weight and Fertility in the Nurses' Health Study

Weight is one bit of information that the participants of the Nurses' Health Study report every other year. By linking this information with their accounts of pregnancy, birth, miscarriage, and difficulty getting pregnant, we were able to see a strong connection between weight and fertility. Women with the lowest and highest BMIs were more likely to have had trouble with ovulatory infertility than women in the middle, as shown in Figure 10.3.[5] Infertility was least common among women with BMIs of 20 to 24, with an ideal around 21.

Keep in mind that this is a statistical model of probabilities that links weight and fertility. It doesn't mean you'll get pregnant only if you have a BMI between 20 and 24. Women with higher and lower BMIs than this get pregnant all the time without delay or any medical help. But it supports the idea that weighing too much or too little for your frame can get in the way of having a baby.

Fertility Zone for Weight

We call the range of BMIs from 20 to 24 the fertility zone. (You can find your BMI by using Figure 10.2.) It isn't magic—nothing is for fertility—but having a weight in that range seems to be best for getting pregnant. If you aren't in or near the zone, don't despair. Working to move your BMI in that direction by gaining or losing some weight is almost as good. Relatively small changes are often enough to have the desired effects of healthy ovulation and improved fertility. If you are too lean, gaining

Table 10.1 **Body Fat and Hormones**

Fat cells, also known as adipocytes, secrete numerous hormones or cell-signaling molecules that affect metabolism, appetite, and other aspects of nutrition. Several of these hormones also affect insulin sensitivity and reproduction, usually in ways that are counterproductive to good health and fertility.

Hormone	Primary Action	Effect of Excess Weight on Hormone Level	Effect on Insulin Sensitivity	Possible Effect on Reproduction
Adiponectin	Increases cells' burning of fat and improves insulin sensitivity	Decreases	Increases	Enhances ovulation
Interleukin-6	Stimulates cell growth	Increases	Decreases	Interferes with implantation of a fertilized egg
Leptin	Communicates information about energy stores	Increases		Interferes with ovulation
Plasminogen activator inhibitor-1	Inhibits the formation of blood clots in arteries	Increases		Interferes with implantation
Resistin	Influences insulin sensitivity	Increases	Decreases	Interferes with ovulation and implantation
Tumor necrosis factor-alpha	Mediates inflammation	Increases	Decreases	Interferes with implantation

Adapted from Gosman GG and colleagues. Obesity and the role of gut and adipose hormones in female reproduction. *Human Reproduction Update* 2006; 12:585-601.

five or ten pounds can sometimes be enough to restart ovulation and menstrual periods. If you are overweight, losing 5 percent to 10 percent of your current weight is often enough to improve ovulation.

Figure 10.3 **The Fertility Zone for Weight**

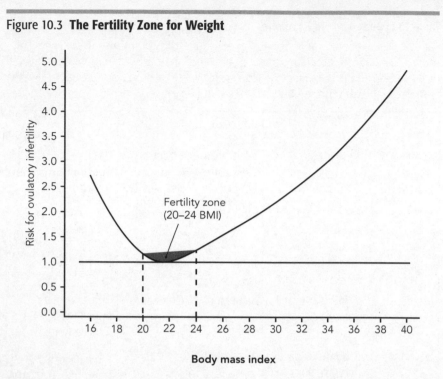

In the Nurses' Health Study, women with BMIs between 20 and 24 were the least likely to have experienced ovulatory infertility. The farther you stray from this fertility zone in either direction, the harder it may be to get pregnant. Being in the zone, or working to move your weight in that direction, can have an enormously positive impact on fertility.

In the pages that follow, we focus on weighing too much, because it is a bigger problem here and around the world. Once considered a problem only in high-income countries like the United States, overweight and obesity are now on the rise in low- and middle-income countries, particularly in urban settings where they often paradoxically stand side by side with malnutrition.

▶The 7½ Percent Solution

Things can look a bit bleak if you are overweight and a healthy weight is many pounds away. Take heart. Numerous studies have shown that overweight women can jump-start ovulation by losing a modest amount of weight—5 to 10 percent of their starting weight—even when that loss doesn't get them into the healthy weight range. It may be a bit less for some, a bit more for others. We'll split the difference and take a middle ground, which we'll call the 7½ percent solution.

Let's put this into practical terms. A 7½ percent weight loss means 12 pounds for a woman starting at 160 pounds, 15 pounds for one starting at 200 pounds, and 19 pounds for one starting at 250 pounds. Although such goals are a challenge, they are far less daunting than "aiming for a healthy weight," the advice usually offered by health care professionals.

Among women with polycystic ovary syndrome (PCOS), this amount of weight loss can not only restore ovulation and menstruation but can also clear the skin and curb excess facial and body hair. These improvements are probably the result of better sensitivity to insulin and a decrease in the amount of male hormones in circulation.

Among *all* overweight women, a modest 7½ percent weight loss improves health across the board. Take prevention of diabetes as an example. A major trial, called the Diabetes Prevention Program, included more than 3,200 people who were at risk for developing type 2 diabetes. Those who lost just 7 percent of their weight and exercised about thirty minutes a day cut their risk of developing diabetes by nearly 60 percent. They decreased their harmful LDL cholesterol and triglyceride levels and increased their protective HDL, sometimes more than people in the study who took metformin, an antidiabetes drug.[6] Losing a modest amount of weight can have positive effects on other "silent" conditions, like high blood pressure or kidney disease.

WHAT IS A POUND?

A pound of fat is the equivalent of 3,500 calories. Burn 3,500 more than you take in and you've lost a pound. Take in 3,500 more than you burn and you've gained a pound—at least to a point. As you gain weight, you add some muscle to support it and spend more energy carrying it around. So the more weight you gain, the more calories it takes to add an extra pound.

It can also make a difference in how you feel, from easing the sleep-stealing breathing problem known as sleep apnea to alleviating arthritis pain and giving you more energy.

Getting to 7½

So how do you attain the 7½ percent solution?

An extraordinarily simple equation describes how to shed pounds:

$$\text{calories out} > \text{calories in} = \text{weight loss}$$

In English: burn more calories than you take in day after day and you will absolutely, positively end up weighing less than when you started.

Of course, Einstein's $e = mc^2$ is also a simple equation. It's too bad that the ease of explaining something doesn't necessarily indicate how easily it can be translated into action.

When it comes to losing weight, creating an imbalance between calories in and calories out isn't as simple as falling off a log. Appetite, metabolism, and life get in the way, making weight loss a challenge for most people and seemingly impossible for some. But you can do it. You have a goal—having a baby—that is a powerful motivator. By following the strategies outlined in this chapter, you can lose weight in a way that is good for your health, fertility, peace of mind, and relationship with food.

Do the Math

Advice gleaned from an ancient Chinese manual on the art of war applies perfectly to the battle of the bulge: "Know your enemy and know yourself; in a hundred battles, you will never be defeated." The key things you need to know about your "enemy" and yourself are:

- What are your eating patterns?
- Are you burning many calories?

Before plunging into a weight-loss program, take the time to gather this information. It will help you figure out how and what to change in your diet and what kind of a boost you will get from exercise.

If you are a woman of action and know you need to lose weight, you can go straight to the "Get Started" section. Read on, however, if you'd like to understand your habits a bit better before making changes.

Tracking Your Eating Pattern. Few of us have a good handle on what we eat each day. Keeping a food log or diary for a few days can give you an idea of what you eat, when, and sometimes why. It can be as simple as a piece of notebook paper with a few columns or as fancy as a spreadsheet. Or try one of the many free and commercial online food diaries that a Google search for "food diary" will retrieve.

As you keep your diary, jot down when you eat and how you are feeling before and afterward. This information can give you a glimpse into your eating patterns, which may sometimes strongly influence what and how much you eat. As a model, we've included a sample one-day food diary in Figure 10.4.

No matter how you keep your diary, *be honest*. Try to list everything you eat and drink. This doesn't just include meals—jot down your snacks, noshes, tastes, and beverages, too.

If you want to tally calories in your food diary, you can. But it isn't necessary. The most important information the diary can reveal is where your calories are coming from. You might find that many of your daily calories are coming from snacks rather than meals, or you are getting a lot of them from dinnertime on instead of spread throughout the day. This can give you an idea as to where you can make the easiest cuts.

Your notes about when you ate and how you were feeling will give you a sense of your eating habits. Did you skimp on breakfast and snack after dinner? Did you eat because you were hungry, bored, or being sociable? After eating, did you feel satisfied, still hungry, or guilty? These can help you identify potential trouble spots when you start cutting back on calories.

If you want to track your calories, that takes a bit of detective work. Any food or snack that comes from a package has its calories listed on the food label. Be careful here. Calories are listed per serving, and some packages contain more than one serving. Serving sizes can be tricky. We've listed examples in "What Counts as a Serving?" Another

Figure 10.4 **Sample Food Diary**

Food Diary			
Food	Time	Feeling?	Calories
Breakfast			
English muffin with butter and jelly	6:45	rushed	268
Mug of coffee with half-and-half and sugar	6:45		112
Snack			
Coffee with milk and sugar, half a bagel	10:00	hungry	60
3 Hershey's Kisses from coworker's stash	11:00		75
Lunch			
Turkey sub with mayonnaise	1:15	hungry, at desk	300
Sprite	1:15	hungry, at desk	96
Small bag of potato chips	1:15	hungry, at desk	310
Snack			
Coffee with milk and sugar	2:30	in a meeting	70
Sprite	4:15	thirsty	96
Apple	5:30	driving home	72
Dinner			
Lasagna (one helping)	7:00	lucky to get dinner on the table	375
Green beans	7:00		35
Bread	7:00		80
Salad with ranch dressing	7:00		80
Glass of red wine	7:00		125
Snack			
Dish of chocolate ice cream	9:30	while watching TV	143
Total			**2,297**

Keeping a simple food diary can give you an idea of your eating patterns. It isn't necessary to track calories to know what to do—if your weight is creeping up, you are eating too much. But if you have the time and interest, the calorie count may come as a motivating surprise.

way to get a food's calorie count is with the National Nutrient Database (www.nal.usda.gov/fnic/foodcomp/search) from the U.S. Department of Agriculture. This free resource is a treasure trove of information on thousands of foods. Say you want to know how many calories are in a three-ounce fillet of sole. Enter "sole" in the keywords box. Choose cooked sole from the list that appears. Check the box for 3 ounces and voilà: more nutritional information about sole than you ever imagined. Calories are listed second, as energy in kcal (short for kilocalories, which are food calories).

WHAT COUNTS AS A SERVING?

Here's how the USDA's Food and Nutrition Service tallies up serving sizes:

Grains
- 1 slice of bread
- 1 cup (about 1 ounce) of ready-to-eat cereal
- ½ cup of cooked cereal, rice, or pasta

Vegetables
- 1 cup of raw leafy vegetables
- ½ cup of other vegetables, cooked or raw
- ¾ cup of vegetable juice

Fruits
- 1 medium apple, banana, or orange
- ½ cup of chopped, cooked, or canned fruit
- ¾ cup of fruit juice

Dairy
- 1 cup of milk or yogurt
- 1½ ounces of natural cheese (like cheddar or Swiss)
- 2 ounces of processed cheese (like American)

Meat and Other Protein Sources
- 2–3 ounces of cooked lean meat, poultry, or fish

These count as 1 ounce of lean meat:

- ½ cup of cooked dry beans
- 2 tablespoons of peanut butter
- 1 egg
- ⅓ cup of nuts

Unfortunately, the federal government doesn't keep serving sizes consistent from agency to agency. The FDA uses different and more complex definitions for serving sizes on food labels. It spells these out for food makers in nine pages of tiny type in the U.S. Code of Federal Regulations.

Source: *The Food Guide Pyramid: A Guide to Daily Food Choices*, U.S. Department of Agriculture, www.nal.usda.gov/fnic/Fpyr/pmap.htm.

At the end of the day, add up the calorie column. You might find you have a good handle on what you are taking in. On the other hand, you might be surprised to see the tally.

Estimating Calories Out. Determining calories burned is a difficult proposition. To get an exact count, you would need to be hooked up to a machine that records how much oxygen you use and how much carbon dioxide you give off all day in a temperature-controlled lab. *That's* certainly not an option. Instead, a little more math can help you estimate the number of calories you need to maintain your current weight. Although this is influenced by your weight, height, age, health, and body composition, you can get a rough idea by multiplying your weight times:

- 12 if you are sedentary (little or no exercise)
- 13.5 if you are somewhat active (light exercise one to three days a week)
- 15.5 if you are moderately active (moderate exercise like brisk walking three to five days a week)
- 17 if you are very active (vigorous exercise or sports six to seven days a week)
- 19 if you are highly active (daily vigorous exercise or sports and a physical job)

For example, a somewhat active woman who weighs 145 pounds needs about 1,950 calories a day (145 times 13.5) to keep a steady weight.

Get Started

Once you understand the ins and outs of your weight, start making some changes. If you are a do-it-yourselfer, go ahead and fiddle with your diet. This isn't rocket science and only you know what foods you like, which ones you can't stand, and what sorts of changes will work for you. The goal is a slow, sensible approach that improves your weight and your fertility. Based on what we have learned from the Nurses' Health Study, this would be a diet rich in plant protein, whole grains, and healthful unsaturated fats; low in refined carbohydrates and in trans and saturated fats; and with a daily serving of whole milk or other full-fat dairy products. The meal plans and recipes in Chapter 13 offer ideas for putting this into practice. We describe how to structure your own weight-loss fertility diet in "Ten Tips for Doing It Yourself."

If you would rather have some guidance, you can turn to any of the hundreds of available diet books, commercial weight-loss plans, self-help organizations, and e-diets. We'll help you sort the wheat from the chaff in "Losing Weight by the Book."

Skipping 250 Calories

The word *diet* usually conjures up images of austerity—plain toast, salad, fat-free cottage cheese, a dry chicken breast. There's really no need for that. You can lose weight with a flavorful, filling diet that includes foods that are good for you and the baby you hope to have.

A consistent body of research shows that the average person can stop her or his natural weight gain by eating one hundred fewer calories a day. Halting weight gain is a great place to start, but it isn't going to calm the hormonal winds that dry up ovulation. There's no need to dramatically slash your food intake, either. Instead, try cutting it

Table 10.2 **Twenty-Five Easy Foods to Avoid with 200 (or More) Calories**

Food	Serving Size	Calories
French fries, McDonald's	1 large order	573
Subway six-inch Steak and Cheese	1	400
Baked potato with sour cream	1 medium	393
Kentucky Fried Popcorn Chicken	4 ounces	370
Cheese Danish	1 medium	353
Eggnog	1 cup	343
Potato chips	2 ounces	310
Starbucks Caffe Mocha, with whole milk and whipped cream	12 ounces	310
Gummy worms	10	293
Chocolate ice cream	1 cup	286
Tortilla chips	2 ounces	274
Taco Bell Chili Cheese Burrito	1	270
Snickers bar	2 ounces	266
Cinnamon coffee cake	2 ounces	263
Plain bagel	4-inch diameter	257
Burger King BK Big Fish Sandwich	1	250
Breakfast sausages	3	247
Piña colada	4½ ounces	245
Hot dog, plain	1 medium	242
Doughnut, raised, plain	1	240
Graham crackers	2 ounces	236
Croissant, plain	1	231
Pretzels, hard	2 ounces	228
Strawberry Pop-Tart (not frosted)	1 pastry	210
Sprite	16-ounce bottle	197

Calorie counts are from the U.S. Department of Agriculture and food company nutrition information. (The USDA offers a free list of the caloric content of nearly 1,200 foods: www.nal.usda.gov/fnic/foodcomp/Data/SR18/nutrlist/sr18w208.pdf.)

by 250 calories a day. That's one can of sugared soda and two regular Oreos, or a two-ounce bag of potato chips. Table 10.2 lists other examples of foods containing 200 or more calories that you could easily do without. With this modest daily reduction in calories, you could lose two pounds a month. Add thirty minutes of brisk walking if you don't already exercise, or ratchet up the pace of your routine if you do, and you could lose three pounds. (Exercise is such an important part of losing weight and improving fertility that we devote the next chapter to it.)

This kind of steady weight loss won't get you on "Oprah" or land you a contract as the poster person for a weight-loss infomercial. It's possible your family and friends might not notice, at least not at first. But your body will. Your tissues will slowly but surely become more sensitive to insulin; exercise speeds this vital process. As your supply of body fat shrinks, so will the gusts of ovulation-interfering hormones that too much body fat constantly wafts into the bloodstream.

A thoughtful, measured approach to losing weight gives you time to acclimate to new habits and new foods. It also lets your body gradually adjust to fewer calories. At some point you may hit a plateau where you won't see much weight loss, even though you are sticking with your plan. What's happening is that your body's metabolism is compensat-

WHERE DOES LOST WEIGHT GO?

You know all too well where the pounds go when you gain weight—usually your thighs, belly, and derriere. Where do they go when you lose weight? Into heat, water, and carbon dioxide, mostly. When you take in fewer calories than your body needs to beat your heart, pump your lungs, circulate blood, think thoughts, and move you from one place to another, your body dips into its energy stores. Fats are burned to support these functions. This conversion yields chemical energy, which your body uses immediately, along with heat, water, and carbon dioxide. You use some of the heat to keep your body warm. Your kidneys remove some of the water and divert it into urine. And you breathe out the carbon dioxide. Though one breath may seem weightless, you actually breathe out more than two pounds of carbon dioxide a day and more when losing weight.

ing for the reduction in calories. When you notice this happening, it's time to start looking to cut back another 250 calories and give your metabolism a kick with more physical activity. By this time, though, you will be in better shape and the extra activity will come easier.

Ten Tips for Doing It Yourself

"Diet book, schmiet book—I can do this myself," you say. And you can. All diet plans work by getting you to take in fewer calories than you burn each day. Some do it through sheer monotony, like the infamous grapefruit diet. Others claim that their special blend of foods revs up your metabolism and makes you burn fat faster. In reality, most diets work by making you more aware of what you are eating, and it is this mindfulness that helps you cut back on calories.

You can build your own slimming diet with the following ten tips. To make it work for fertility as well as for weight loss, keep it rich in plant protein, whole grains, and healthful unsaturated fats and low in refined carbohydrates as well as trans and saturated fats, and have a serving of whole milk or other full-fat dairy food every day. And make sure you support it with more than thirty minutes of exercise a day.

1. Eat a good breakfast within a couple hours of waking up. Good choices include an egg, yogurt, or oatmeal, with whole wheat toast on the side.
2. Have at least two *extra* servings a day of nonstarchy vegetables (like asparagus, beets, broccoli, carrots, cauliflower, cucumbers, green beans, tomatoes, zucchini, and any green, leafy vegetable), for a total of at least five vegetable servings. Don't include potatoes as a vegetable.
3. Have at least one *extra* serving a day of a low-sugar fruit (like apples, berries, citrus fruits, melon, mango, papaya, peaches, and plums), for a total of at least three fruit servings.
4. When choosing carbohydrates, go for whole grains. Limit your easily digested starches (like white bread, white rice, and potatoes) to once a day.

5. Have some protein at every meal. Whenever possible, choose plant protein (like beans and nuts) or fish.

6. Focus on healthy fats. Fats, like protein, help you feel full longer. They also slow the digestion of carbohydrates. Make sure to choose healthful unsaturated fats, like olive and canola oils. Cut back on saturated fats and avoid trans fats.

7. If you enjoy sweets or dessert, don't kill yourself avoiding them. Treat yourself every other day with something your taste buds will look forward to, like a small bowl of ice cream, a sugar-free Fudgsicle, three Hershey's Kisses, or a small square of rich, dark chocolate. Savor it!

8. Try to drink at least forty-eight ounces of water (tea and coffee count) every day. Take sugared soda and fruit drinks off your menu. If you need to sip a sweet, fizzy drink, make it a diet soda.

9. Try not to eat anything after dinner.

10. Add a prenatal vitamin for insurance.

Losing Weight by the Book

If you could read a book a day, you might be able to wade through the new diet books published last year. Not that you'd want to, of course. In addition to sitting for so long—and probably gaining weight in the process—you would go crazy from the contradicting claims and approaches. Eat carbs. Avoid flour. Melt away fat. End your diet war and achieve thinner peace. Lose weight by eating in reverse—breakfast for dinner and vice versa. Let coconut help you lose weight. Eat like a caveman or cavewoman. Get God on your team and lose weight as the Bible taught. Hypnotize yourself slimmer. The list goes on.

The staggering amount of diet advice available in books new and old is enough to make you shy away from picking one. That's one reason why people tend to try diets they've heard about or those with a media buzz. Think of the Atkins sensation or the Scarsdale diet. They worked (for some people) but eventually faded from prominence, to be replaced by the next big thing.

) FAD DIET OR BAD DIET?

No matter what the books or ads say, there is no such thing as an easy way to lose weight. Pounds don't melt away—you work them away. Be leery of any weight-loss program that:

- Promises you'll lose more than two pounds a week. It's possible to do that but not safe. Weight lost that fast usually reappears just as quickly.
- Says you don't need to exercise or change your eating habits. You'll need both to lose weight and, more important, to keep it off.
- Relies on "miracle" foods, supplements, body wraps, creams, etc. Hype to the contrary, no foods or food extracts have yet been discovered that make fat vanish.
- Requires you to eat just one food or a limited number of them. The cabbage soup diet might work for a few days, but you'll be eating something else, perhaps without regard for your weight, within a short time.
- Sounds too good to be true. It is.

Almost any diet book can help you shed a few pounds. What you need is a sensible approach that will guide you to eat a healthful, balanced diet that's good for fertility, pregnancy, and long-term health. That's a tall order. Here are some suggestions on how various popular diets can and can't help.

Low-Fat Diets

Examples: *Eat More, Weigh Less; The Pritikin Principle*
Trading on the theories that eating fat makes you fat and that fat is bad for the heart, a host of books try to squeeze out the fat from your diet. Unfortunately, neither of those notions is true. Some fats are good for the heart, and a diet with a moderate amount of healthy fats can promote weight loss as well as, or better than, low-fat diets.

Because carbohydrate and protein contain just four calories per gram, compared to nine calories per gram for fat, you can actually eat more food by switching from fatty foods to carbohydrate-rich ones, especially fruits and vegetables. That's a plus. The problem for many people is that low-fat diets tend to be lean on flavor, because fats make foods taste good. Low-fat diets can also leave you feeling hungry, which is why they usually call for high-fiber foods, which increase the sensation of fullness, as well as between-meal snacks.

If you choose a low-fat approach, be sure to include whole-grain options when the diet calls for bread, pasta, or other grains.

Low-Carb Diets

Examples: *Dr. Atkins' New Diet Revolution; The South Beach Diet*

Although the Atkins and South Beach diets may have given the low-carb approach a huge new audience, blaming carbohydrates as the culprit of unwanted pounds isn't new. In 1863, British carpenter and undertaker William Banting published his *Letter on Corpulence*. In it he described his twenty-year quest to lose weight and how he methodically lost fifty pounds over the course of a year by giving up bread, butter, milk, sugar, beer, potatoes, and other sweets and starches. In its day, Banting's *Letter* was as popular as the Atkins and South Beach diets.

There's actually some good science to back up the notion that high-protein, low-carbohydrate diets work for weight loss. Three factors play different roles. Chicken, beef, fish, beans, and other high-protein foods slow the movement of food from the stomach to the intestine, which means you feel full longer and get hungrier later. Protein has a gentler, steadier effect on blood sugar, which helps avoid the steep rise and rapid fall in blood sugar and insulin that occur after eating a rapidly digested carbohydrate like white bread or baked potato. And it takes more energy to digest protein than it does to break down carbohydrates.

The biggest controversy with low-carb diets is what to eat in place of refined carbohydrates. The early Atkins diet banned carbohydrates in virtually every form and gloried in hamburgers, steak, sausage, cheese, and other foods rich in saturated fat. The latest Atkins diet allows some carbohydrates—mainly fruits, vegetables, and some whole grains—after an initial no-carb period. The South Beach diet, which also promotes protein and counsels cutting back on carbohydrates, takes a harder line against bad fats.

If you go the low-carb route, choose your protein wisely. Options such as fish, beans, and nuts are better than steak and sausage. And think twice about shying away completely from whole grains, fruits, and vegetables. They give you vitamins, minerals, fiber, and phytonutrients you just can't get anywhere else.

Correct-Carb Diets

Examples: *The Glucose Revolution; The New Sugar Busters*

An interesting variation on low-carb diets are correct-carb diets, which advise eating by the glycemic index, a measure of how fast the body digests the carbohydrate in different foods. (We described this in more detail in Chapter 4.) The idea behind correct-carb diets is that choosing foods with a low glycemic index helps you avoid the blood sugar rush and crash that you get with foods made with highly refined grains, such as white bread, most bagels, white rice, and potatoes. The right carbs include beans, most fruits and vegetables, and whole grains.

Carefully choosing your carbohydrates is a fine idea for weight loss, fertility, and general health. But the glycemic index is just one factor that will help you choose carbohydrates that will fill you up without causing a sugar rush. Focusing on foods higher in fiber, even if the glycemic index is moderate, is also important.

Perfect Proportions and Correct Combinations

Examples: *The Zone; Eat Right 4 Your Type*

One idea that comes and goes in diet books is that specific proportions of nutrients or combinations of foods are keys to weight loss. To get into the Zone, which is supposed to be a state of near-perfect insulin production, you need to create meals and snacks with the magic ratio of 40 percent/30 percent/30 percent, or nine grams of carbohydrate for every seven grams of protein and one-and-a-half grams of fat. *Eat Right 4 Your Type* says that your blood type determines what you should eat, how you should exercise, what supplements you need, and what type of personality you have. Good luck having a family dinner if there are four of you with different blood types. So far, there isn't any evidence that Zone-like proportions or blood-type combinations work any better than other diets. Any success they have is mainly because they help you focus on what you are eating and eat less each day.

Calorie Density
Example: *Volumetrics*

This plan, developed by respected nutrition researcher Barbara Rolls, focuses on foods that fill you up without adding too many calories. It encourages you to eat foods with a high water content—fruits, vegetables, low-fat milk, cooked grains, beans, soups, and stews. High-fat foods, which pack a lot of calories, and dry, calorie-dense ones, like pretzels, crackers, and fat-free cookies, get the thumbs-down. There are exceptions. Some foods with very high energy densities, like nuts, are very satisfying, and people who regularly eat nuts don't tend to weigh more than those who don't eat nuts. It is possible that calorie density may influence body weight, but so far there isn't any evidence from long-term studies that a low-density diet is effective for weight loss.

Although you could adopt a relatively healthful diet by following the Volumetrics plan, it can be awfully lean. Don't ignore healthful unsaturated fats just because they have more calories per gram than fruits and vegetables. Unsaturated fats may improve fertility, are good for long-term health, and, as Mediterranean and other diets show, can be part of a successful weight-loss plan.

Behavior Change
Examples: *The Ultimate Weight Solution; The Automatic Diet*

Some people use food for comfort and overeat in response to sadness, loneliness, depression, or any number of other triggers. Various diet books aim to help you break unhealthy relationships with food. Some get you to think about when and why you eat. Others use behavior modification techniques to reprogram the patterns that work against healthy eating. Such approaches aren't for everyone. But if you think that your habits, behaviors, and/or relationships with other people—and with food—are keeping you from a healthy weight, then a behavioral approach makes sense. Combining it with a healthy eating pattern based on sound nutrition would be even better.

Mediterranean Style

Examples: *The Mediterranean Diet; Eat, Drink, & Weigh Less; The Sonoma Diet*

In the 1950s and 1960s, pioneering nutrition researcher Ancel Keys and his colleagues found that people living in Crete, other parts of Greece, and southern Italy lived longer and had less heart disease than their counterparts in similar countries. Keys concluded from what came to be known as the Seven Countries Study that the traditional diet was an important reason for this. At the time, the traditional diet in these Mediterranean regions included mostly plant-based foods—fruits, vegetables, breads, coarsely ground grains, beans, nuts, and seeds. Olive oil was the main source of dietary fat. People regularly ate dairy products, mostly cheese and yogurt, but not in large amounts. Poultry and red meat were eaten on special occasions, not as part of the daily fare. Wine was typically drunk with meals.

Keys and his wife, Margaret, published *How to Eat Well and Stay Well the Mediterranean Way* in 1975. Since then, other books have promoted this traditional diet as a way to lose weight and stay healthy. They emphasize good fats and good carbs, variety, plenty of fruits and vegetables, and moderation.

Over the years, researchers have accumulated strong evidence that both the traditional diet and the traditional lifestyle—lots of exercise and physical activity, regular meal patterns, relatively little stress, and wine—contributed to the unusually good health of those living in Crete and the nearby regions that Ancel Keys and company investigated. In one of the few rigorous comparison studies of different diets, Kathy McManus and her colleagues at Harvard-affiliated Brigham and Women's Hospital found that a Mediterranean-type diet is good for long-term weight loss. They randomly assigned 101 overweight volunteers to either a low-fat (20 percent fat) diet or a moderate-fat (35 percent) Mediterranean-type diet that included an abundance of vegetables, nuts, and whole grains flavored richly with herbs and olive oil. At six months, both groups had similar and impressive weight loss. After that, though, volunteers in the low-fat group began regaining weight, and most dropped out of the study. Those who stuck with the low-fat diet had regained most of their weight by eighteen months. In contrast, those following the Mediterranean-type diet kept off the pounds they had shed. At eighteen months, more than half were still sticking with the diet, and many maintained their weight loss even at thirty months. One reason for its success was that the participants said they didn't feel deprived and were very satisfied with the variety and flavors of their new way of eating.[7]

The variety of a Mediterranean-type diet, as well as its emphasis on good carbs, good fats, and good protein, make it a generally good choice for fertility as well.

Programming Weight Loss

Books, of course, aren't the only source of how-to information on losing weight. A host of programs have been developed to help people shed pounds. Two of the most popular are Weight Watchers and Jenny Craig. These commercial programs focus on balanced low-fat, low-calorie nutrition that can lead to modest (a pound or two a week) weight loss. Although they use different strategies for cutting calories, both help with the initial stage of weight loss. But they don't necessarily teach dieters how to manage their intake of food, or prepare healthful foods, over the long term. Another popular program is eDiets. This online service provides information and support for following a variety of different diets.

One of the big advantages of programs like these is the support they offer dieters, something that isn't generally available from diet books. This support, from trained counselors or other dieters, helps some people stick with their weight-loss strategies longer than they would have without the help.

Head-to-Head Comparisons

One of the things that makes recommending diet books difficult is the dearth of research on the diets they promote. There's no law that says you have to test a diet before writing a book about it. All you need is an idea and a way to promote it. Few diets have ever been put to any kind of rigorous test, and there are even fewer head-to-head studies.

Most direct comparisons suggest that it isn't the diet plan that makes a difference but whether you stick with it. In a 2005 study published in the *Journal of the American Medical Association*, researchers randomly assigned 160 overweight and obese adults to one of four popular diet plans: the Atkins diet, the Ornish diet, Weight Watchers, and the Zone diet. After one year, nearly half of the participants had dropped out. But those who completed the study lost similar amounts of weight (an average of five to seven pounds each).[8] They also lowered their blood levels of cholesterol and improved other markers linked to heart disease and diabetes to a similar degree. People assigned to the Atkins and Ornish diets were more likely to drop out of the study, suggesting that many people found these plans too extreme.

A similar comparison, published two years later in the same prestigious journal, compared weight loss over the course of a year among 311 overweight but healthy women assigned to one of four diets: Atkins, Zone, Ornish, or the Lifestyles, Exercise, Attitudes, Relationships, and Nutrition (LEARN) plan, a standard low-fat, moderately high-carbohydrate diet. Although the women in all four groups steadily lost weight for the first six months, the most rapid weight loss occurred among the Atkins dieters. After that, most of the participants started to regain weight. At the end of a year, it looked as though the women in the Atkins group had lost the most weight, about ten pounds, compared to where they had started, compared with almost six pounds for the LEARN group, five for the Ornish group, and three and a half for the Zone group.[9] The fine print of the study, though, revealed that few of the women actually stuck with their assigned diets. Those in the Atkins group were aiming for fifty grams of carbohydrate a day but took in almost triple that amount. The Ornish dieters were supposed to limit their fat intake to under 10 percent of their daily calories but got about 30 percent from fat. There were similar deviations for the Zone and LEARN groups.

In both studies, the overall results mask startling individual differences. In the 2005 trial, for example, some people lost weight and some gained weight on both low-carb and low-fat diets. In the low-fat group, the range was from fifty-three pounds lost to thirty-one pounds gained. In the low-carb group, it was from sixty-five pounds lost to eighteen gained.[8]

There are several take-home messages from these and other head-to-head diet comparisons. The first is that one type of nutrient isn't necessarily better than another—you can lose weight with any diet that helps you eat less. Finding strategies that help you match your food intake to the calories you burn matters far more than focusing on macronutrients like protein, fat, or carbohydrates. Another equally important lesson is that it is OK to experiment on yourself. If you give a diet your best shot and it doesn't work, maybe it wasn't the right one for you, your metabolism, or your situation. Don't get too discouraged or beat yourself up because a diet that "worked for everybody" didn't pay off for you. Try another. Keep in mind, though, that your real goal isn't a quick and temporary fix. Instead, try to find a way of eating that delivers foods and nutrients that will make your life a long and enjoyable one and that also helps you control your weight.

▶ Fat Doesn't Make You Fat

Whether you are trying to cut calories on your own or with the help of a diet book, it is tempting to focus on fats. After all, one gram of fat has nine calories. That's more than twice as many calories per gram as for protein or carbohydrate, which have four each. And there's a lovely logic to the notion that eating fat makes you fat, so avoiding dietary fat will slim you down. If that were the case, we'd be a trimmer nation. Over the past couple decades, as a nation we have cut our fat intake from 40 percent of calories to around 33 percent. Yet this was accompanied by an increase in weight and a dramatic rise in obesity.

Low fat doesn't mean low calorie. Some fat-free foods actually contain more calories than the regular versions because the manufacturers use extra sugar to make up for the taste that was lost with the fat. Adding insult to injury, many low-fat foods are made by removing healthful unsaturated fats.

The trick is to be selective. By all means cut back on saturated and trans fats. Neither of these are good for your arteries or your hopes for having a baby. As we described in Chapter 5, trans fats pose a particular hazard for ovulation. But don't shy away from healthful unsaturated fats in salad dressings, fish, nuts, avocados, and oils like olive and canola oil.

▶Beware of Liquid Calories

When trying to cut calories, don't overlook what you are drinking. Beverages are an often invisible source of calories, mostly empty ones that are devoid of vitamins, minerals, fiber, and other nutrients. A standard twelve-ounce can of sugared soda or bottle of juice delivers 150 to 200 calories. A large one (thirty-two ounces) gives you more than 300 calories. Many people drink juice because they think that it is good for them. That might be true for a small glass at breakfast, but having juice the rest of the day isn't a good idea. Tea and coffee by themselves have no calories. Add a stream of cream and two sugars, and zero becomes 60—or more. A large Starbucks White Chocolate Frappuccino with whipped cream, for example, delivers the caloric equivalent of a full though unhealthy meal, with 760 calories and thirteen grams of saturated fat. Alcoholic drinks are another source of hidden calories. The average glass of wine or bottle of beer contains between 100 and 150 calories.

Another problem with liquid calories is that people don't always compensate for what they take in with beverages. An innovative study from Purdue University bears this out. Fifteen healthy men and women were asked to take in an extra 450 calories a day for four weeks. Some did this by eating jelly beans, others by drinking sugared soda. After two weeks, the soda drinkers switched to jelly beans and the jelly bean eaters switched to soda. Over the course of the study, the jelly bean eaters reduced the number of calories they took in from other sources and gained only a small amount of weight. The soda drinkers didn't make adjustments and gained much more weight.[10]

As we describe in Chapter 9, water is best for quenching your thirst. If plain water is too, well, plain, try fizzy water or add a slice of lemon, lime, or orange or a sprig of mint.

▶Good Habits Help

While cutting calories and exercising more are the stars when it comes to losing weight, you need a strong supporting cast for a long, successful run. These include behaviors and habits that can help you avoid the environmental and psychological factors that may have led to the weight gain in the first place and that often make it tough to sustain a diet or exercise routine. Many of the following strategies seem like common sense, but they are easily overlooked. You will be most likely to follow them if you plan for them in advance.

■ **Slow down.** Chewing and swallowing your food at a leisurely pace can help keep you from overeating. Here's why: it takes a few minutes for your stomach's "I'm getting full" signal to get to your brain. Eating slowly gives your brain the time it needs to signal the rest of you that you've had enough.

■ **Ease into it.** Instead of switching overnight to a lower-calorie eating plan, try phasing it in. Start by cutting out snacking or limiting yourself to certain snacks at certain times of day (such as a midmorning handful of nuts or a late-afternoon apple). Then lower the calorie content of one meal at a time. In the first week, try eating a lower-calorie lunch, but keep breakfast and dinner the same as before. During the second week, reduce the calorie content of your dinner. Finally, you can cut some calories from your breakfast. Don't skimp too much on breakfast, though. Tempting though that might be, you usually end up paying for it with rushed, midmorning high-calorie snacks. Be sure your meals contain some protein, slow carbs, and unsaturated fats. That will make snacks less urgent and less necessary.

■ **Keep track.** A daily log of what you eat and your physical activity can help keep you motivated to stay with your diet and exercise plan. A week's worth of entries can tell you how successful you've been and help you identify trouble spots. Weigh yourself weekly so you know how you are doing.

■ **Seek support.** Dieting can sometimes feel like a you-against-the-world endeavor. That isolation makes it harder to change your environment and maintain the changes you need in order to lose weight. It's easier if you have the support and encouragement of others. Enlist your family to eat the same meals you do. Ask them to keep high-calorie foods out of the house (or at least refrain from eating them in front of you). Find an exercise buddy, an important key for sticking with an exercise routine. Join a weight-loss support group, either one that meets face-to-face or a virtual one online. The camaraderie can keep your spirits up during the inevitable periods when you become discouraged with your progress.

■ **Follow the list.** Make a list before you go grocery shopping and stick to it. Steer clear of the chip and soda aisles or other areas with the kinds of high-calorie foods you need to avoid.

■ **Out of sight, out of mind.** Put the most tempting foods high up in the cupboard, at the very back of the fridge, or in other inconvenient spots. If you eat them, don't buy more. Better yet, get them out of the house altogether. Replace the cookie jar and candy bowl with a fruit bowl.

■ **Split it up.** Don't eat chips, crackers, or other snacks directly out of a large package. Instead, put a handful into a small bowl—the smaller the better, since it makes the serving look larger—and put the package away.

■ **Restaurant restraint.** Eat a low-calorie snack before going out for a celebration. You're less likely to overindulge if you aren't starving when looking over the menu. Go elsewhere for after-dinner coffee so you are less tempted to segue right into dessert.

■ **Plan for special occasions.** Decide how much you think you should eat before an event, and do your best to stick with that plan. Set some limits before you go to a party, the movies, or watch the Super Bowl. It's frighteningly easy to munch mindlessly.

■ **Find some stress busters.** If you tend to eat too much when things aren't going right, find a way to ease stress that works for you, like meditation, a relaxation technique, listening to music, exercising, or talking to a friend.

What About Supplements, Drugs, and Surgery?

The marketplace is chock-full of weight-loss aids. They range from sleazy "miracle cures" to carefully evaluated medications and operations. No one needs the purported miracle cures, even though millions of people try them. Prescription medications can help guide weight loss in the short-term, but their use during pregnancy (or just prior to it) is not recommended. For women who are extremely overweight, weight-loss surgery can indeed lead to positive changes in weight and insulin resistance, but it is not yet recommended as a way to improve fertility.

Don't Bother with Supplements

Advertising claims for over-the-counter weight-loss remedies make shedding pounds sound simple. The allure of melting away fat with a pill, slapping on a "diet patch" and letting it do all the work, or losing ten pounds over the weekend without dieting or working out is hard to resist. But resist you should. There isn't a shred of scientific proof that they work despite what the ads say. What's more, few if any of these supplements have been tested for safety. Take ephedra as an example. This herbal extract, touted as an effective weight-loss supplement, was implicated in at least ten deaths—including that of twenty-three-year-old Steve Bechler, a prospective pitcher for the Baltimore Orioles—and even more cases of permanent disability before the FDA finally banned products containing ephedra in 2004. Products that have sprung up to replace them—things like Hoodia, bitter orange, and mangosteen—are equally unknown. A poorly thought out law, the 1994 Dietary Supplement Health and Education Act, lets companies sell supplements made from plants and other natural products without having to show that they are effective or safe.

New York Times health columnist Jane Brody hit the nail on the head when she wrote: "Before spending another cent on yet another nonprescription weight-loss remedy, ask yourself: 'If there really was a miracle drug out there, wouldn't it drive out the competition? And wouldn't everyone know about it?' You shouldn't have to go online or ask a store clerk about it."

If companies pushing weight-loss supplements know little about how they affect weight loss and general health, they know less about how they affect fertility and pregnancy. Ephedra was known to cross the placenta and increase fetal heart rate, as well as stimulate uterine contractions, which could cause an abortion or trigger premature labor. How other supplements might affect fertility or a developing baby are a huge unknown.

Uncertainty About Prescription Weight-Loss Drugs and Pregnancy

Over the years, a handful of more rigorously tested drugs have been approved to help people lose weight. Early ones were stimulants that suppress the appetite. Some of these are still available, including phendimetrazine (Bontril), methamphetamine (Desoxyn), and phentermine (Ionamin and Adipex-P). The FDA approved these drugs for short-term use only, meaning a few weeks. That's because they generally don't cause weight loss beyond several weeks, and they can become addictive.

A newer drug called sibutramine (Meridia) helps reduce food intake by acting on the brain's appetite control center. By blocking the action of two brain chemicals, serotonin and norepinephrine, sibutramine can help people feel full with less food and may prolong that feeling. It has been approved for longer use, up to two years.

Orlistat (Xenical) aids weight loss in yet another way. It blocks the intestines from absorbing and digesting some of the fat from food. This undigested fat exits the body via bowel movements. A lower-dose, over-the-counter version known as Alli is now available. Like Meridia, Xenical and Alli have the green light for longer-term use.

Neither sibutramine nor orlistat work miracles. They don't melt pounds away on their own. Take them without cutting calories and exercising and you are likely to reap the side effects without the benefits. And their contribution to weight loss is modest. In a study of orlistat that included nearly five hundred obese volunteers, those who were randomly assigned to take orlistat along with a weight-loss diet had shed an average of nineteen pounds after a year, while those assigned to take a dummy pill and follow the same diet lost about thirteen pounds. In the study's second year, among those who started out on orlistat, those who continued to take the drug regained an average of seven pounds while those who were given an identical placebo pill regained twelve pounds.

Another problem with orlistat is that it blocks *all* fats, including the healthful unsaturated fats that may help you get pregnant and that are essential for the early development of the baby you hope to conceive.

The other big problem with weight-loss medications is that they haven't been carefully tested in women who are trying to become pregnant or those who are pregnant. Neither sibutramine nor orlistat is recommended for use during pregnancy. We think that should apply to women who are trying to become pregnant, too, since it's easy to be pregnant for a few weeks without knowing it.

Surgery

For people with severe obesity, an operation to shrink or bypass the stomach can be an option when diet, exercise, and medications don't work. The long-term results of these procedures, all covered under the term *bariatric surgery*, are pretty impressive. Many people who have bariatric surgery manage to keep off substantial amounts of weight for ten years or more. In the process, type 2 diabetes, sleep apnea, high blood pressure, and other conditions associated with obesity often fade away or even disappear.

Surgery isn't for everyone, of course. It is a substantial procedure that carries short-term risks like infection and even death. It requires lifelong medical monitoring and major changes in diet and lifestyle. And it carries long-term risks like gallstones, kidney stones, ulcers, and something called the dumping syndrome after high-carbohydrate meals, a reaction that causes flushing, sweating, severe fatigue, nausea, vomiting, diarrhea, and intestinal gas. Given the potential for trouble, surgery is recommended only for people who need it the most—those with a body mass index above 40 or those with a body mass index above 35 accompanied by a serious medical condition such as diabetes, obesity-related degeneration of the heart muscle, or severe sleep apnea.

Because excess weight often blocks ovulation, and weight loss can often restore it, there has been some interest in the use of stomach banding or gastric bypass to reverse infertility in women who are severely overweight. So far, there's no clear message from the few small trials that have explored this possibility. Although there are hints that weight-loss surgery may improve fertility, how well a surgically reorganized digestive system sustains both mother and baby during pregnancy is an open question.

The American Society for Reproductive Medicine hasn't yet taken a position on the use of weight-loss surgery for fertility. Until more is known about the safety, side effects, and effectiveness of these procedures with regard to fertility and pregnancy, it's probably too early to do this just to get pregnant when there are safer ways to accomplish your goal.

▶Weight Affects Fertility in Men, Too

As we have mentioned in other chapters, dietary and lifestyle contributions to fertility and infertility in men have received short shrift. Weight is one area in which there has been some research. A few small studies indicate that overweight men aren't as fertile as their healthy-weight counterparts. Excess weight can lower testosterone levels, throw off the ratio of testosterone to estrogen (men make some estrogen, just as women make some testosterone), and hinder the production of sperm cells that are good swimmers. A study published in 2006 of more than two thousand American farmers and their wives showed that as body mass index went up, fertility declined.[11]

In men, the connection between increasing weight and decreasing fertility can't yet be classified as rock solid. But it is good enough to warrant action, mainly because from a health perspective there aren't any downsides to losing weight if you are overweight. We can't define a fertility zone for weight in men, nor can anyone else. In lieu of that, we can say to men who are carrying too many pounds that shedding some could be good for fertility and will be good for overall health. How many pounds? The same 7½ percent solution that works for women will probably pay off for men as well.

▶Pregnancy Weight Watch

Being at a healthy weight or aiming toward one is great for ovulatory function and your chances of getting pregnant. The "side effects" aren't so bad, either. Working to achieve a healthy weight can improve your sensitivity to insulin, your cholesterol, your blood pressure, and your kidney function. It can give you more energy and make you look and feel better.

If you are overweight and getting to a healthy weight looks like an impossible journey, even small changes in the right direction will improve your fertility and overall health. Cutting back by 250 calories a day is an attainable target. Making small changes, like giving up sugared sodas, juices, and other calorie-containing beverages, is an easy first step.

There is no magic diet for weight loss. Whether you choose a do-it-yourself approach or a by-the-book strategy is a matter of personal taste. Either way, try to find a plan that satisfies your appetite while helping you cut back on your daily food intake. Pick one that you are likely to follow for the long run rather than something you will get tired of in a few weeks. Restrictive diets—those that advocate eating only one particular food or avoiding certain food types, like carbohydrates or fat—tend to get monotonous, while those that promote healthful variety are easier to stick with. Finally, adding thirty to sixty minutes of exercise every day is an integral part of any weight-loss plan. We explore this in more detail in the next chapter.

Chapter 11
· · · · · · · · ·

You've Got to Move It, Move It

Baby, we were born to run. That isn't just the tagline of Bruce Springsteen's anthem to young love and leavin' town. It's also a perfect motto for getting pregnant and for living a long, healthy life.

Each of us comes into this life kicking, flailing, and squalling. Toddlers and children are, by nature, always on the move. Adults should be, too, though most of us aren't. That's a problem. Inactivity deprives muscles of the constant push and pull they need to stay healthy. It also saps their ability to respond to insulin and to efficiently absorb blood sugar. When that leads to too much blood sugar and insulin in the bloodstream, it endangers ovulation, conception, and pregnancy.

Physical activity and exercise are the best ways to keep blood sugar and insulin in check, not to mention control weight, strengthen the heart and lungs, build bone, and improve scads of other aspects of health. Physical activity and exercise are recommended and even prescribed for almost everyone—except women who are having trouble getting pregnant. Forty-year-old findings that too much exercise can turn off menstruation and ovulation make some women shy away from exercise and nudge some doctors to recommend avoiding exercise altogether, at least temporarily. That's clearly the right approach for women who exercise hard for many hours a week and who are extremely lean. But taking it easy isn't likely to help women who aren't active or those whose weights are normal or above where they should be. In other words, the vast majority of women.

Some exciting results from the Nurses' Health Study and a handful of small studies show that exercise can be a boon for fertility. These important findings are establishing a vital link between activity and getting pregnant.

In this chapter, we describe why the body needs activity and how it improves fertility and general health, and we present a plan of exercise and activity that is good for both.

Exercise Is Essential, Not Extra

If you have ever broken a bone and had it immobilized in a cast, you know firsthand just how much your muscles need daily activity—when the cast came off, the muscles underneath were probably withered and weak. They wasted away because they weren't used.

EXERCISE OR ACTIVITY?

What's the difference between physical activity and exercise? Both involve three Ms: movement, muscles, and metabolism. Physical activity is the big tent. It covers any movement that involves muscle contractions and an increase in metabolism. This includes everything from housework to marathon running. Exercise is a specific kind of physical activity—one done purposely to improve health and physical fitness. Both exercise and physical activity are good for you, especially when both are part of most, if not all, of your days. Of course, you win in multiple ways when you combine exercise with your daily activities, like walking or riding a bike to work. You not only improve your health (and fertility), but you also reduce your transportation costs, possibly save time, and contribute to a healthier environment by reducing pollution and global warming.

A now-classic experiment called the Dallas Bedrest and Training Study revealed just how quickly and dramatically this happens.[1] In the summer of 1966, five healthy young men spent three weeks of their summer vacations in bed. They weren't lazy or depressed or staging an antiwar protest. Instead, they stayed horizontal twenty-four hours a day for twenty-one days in the name of science. When the men finally got out of bed, they were very weak. Each had a higher heart rate, higher blood pressure, and more body fat, along with less muscle and a weaker heart than he had started out with. It was as if the men had aged twenty years in just three weeks. The volunteers then embarked on an intense eight-week exercise program. It not only reversed the deterioration brought on by bed rest but actually made some of the young men more fit than they had been before the study.

Thirty years later, the researchers tracked down the five men and asked for their help with a follow-up experiment. All agreed. As you might expect, they had put on some weight (an average of fifty pounds) and had a higher proportion of body fat to muscle, and the pumping power of their hearts had declined. A six-month program of walking, jogging, and cycling seemed to turn back the clock, at least as far as their hearts were concerned: their heart rates, blood pressure, and maximum pumping power returned to what they had been before their three weeks of bed rest.[2]

An updated version of the study, this one including a dozen older men and women (average age, sixty-seven years) showed the same thing, only worse—the participants lost more muscle in ten days than the younger men lost in a month. Leg muscles were the hardest hit.[3]

Those are clear examples of the hazards of inactivity and the restorative power of exercise. A daily swim, run, brisk walk, or Pilates class is the closest thing you have to a magic bullet for preventing or controlling heart disease, diabetes, osteoporosis, and a host of other physical woes. A landmark report from the U.S. Surgeon General, *Physical Activity and Health*,[4] says that exercise and physical activity:

- Improve your chances of living longer and living healthier
- Help protect you from developing heart disease or its handmaidens, high blood pressure and high cholesterol

- Help protect you from developing certain cancers, including colon and breast cancer
- Help prevent type 2 diabetes
- Help prevent the insidious bone loss known as osteoporosis
- Help prevent arthritis and relieve pain and stiffness in people with this condition
- Reduce the risk of falling among older adults
- Relieve symptoms of depression and anxiety and improve mood
- Help prevent impotence
- Control weight

Fertility isn't on this list, but it should be. Chalk up its omission to a series of studies that warned of the possible danger of excessive exercise in a specific—and very small—group of women.

Mixed Messages

In the 1970s, Harvard reproductive biologist Rose E. Frisch began studying highly active women, like young ballet dancers and elite college athletes. As she details in her delightful book *Female Fertility and the Body Fat Connection*,[5] rigorous daily training and strict weight control can delay menarche, the age of first menstruation. In women who are already menstruating when they take up dance or sports, it can halt monthly periods. This certainly didn't happen to all of the dancers or female athletes she studied or even to most of them. Instead, it was most common among those who needed—or wanted—to keep their weight low, such as gymnasts, swimmers, long-distance runners, and lightweight rowers. For these women, stopping daily workouts or gaining a small amount of weight was often all it took to jump-start menstruation.

In Dr. Frisch's view, the main culprit wasn't exercise but an inadequate supply of stored energy. The young women she studied were extremely lean, with little body fat. Many had body mass indexes (BMIs) under 18.

Short-term trials in which healthy, normal-weight, normally menstruating women were asked to exercise very vigorously for a few weeks bear out these findings. Abnormal menstrual bleeding or hormonal changes likely to cause infertility were more pronounced in women who lost a substantial amount of weight as they exercised.[6]

The combination of heavy exercise and leanness interferes with the hypothalamus's ability to generate gonadotropin-releasing hormone. As production of this key reproductive hormone falters, so does the pituitary gland's production of luteinizing hormone. Because luteinizing hormone is needed to make eggs mature and to prepare the endometrium to receive a fertilized egg, turning off the supply of luteinizing hormone derails ovulation and the body's multifaceted preparation for pregnancy. This makes sense from a survival point of view. When the body senses that it doesn't have enough stored energy to sustain a pregnancy, it shuts down the reproductive system rather than investing an immense amount of energy in a pregnancy that would likely fail and might also impair the mother's survival.

This can be seen in the dramatic fall in fertility that accompanied the Dutch famine at the end of World War II, which we describe in Chapter 10.[7] It is also the genesis of more natural fertility cycles. Native Americans living along the Pacific coast in what is now Washington and Oregon, for example, were once fertile during the salmon runs, when there was plenty to eat, but not during the rest of the year, when food was scarce. A similar pattern exists in the hill country of India and agricultural regions of Bangladesh and Gambia, where birth rates follow a seasonal pattern, hitting a peak about nine months after the harvest season.[5,8]

▶Nurses Say "Go"

The work of Dr. Frisch and others sounded a warning about the reproductive consequences of excessive exercise and leanness. But what about more usual amounts of exercise among women who aren't too lean or who don't normally exercise? Is it a hazard for them, too?

Those crucial questions were the focus of a project by one of our colleagues, Janet Rich-Edwards. She looked at physical activity and ovulatory function in the Nurses' Health Study. Of the twenty-six thousand women in her study, the majority reported getting less than an hour of vigorous activity a week. Vigorous activities included jogging, cycling, aerobic dancing, tennis or squash, and other pursuits listed in "Moderate or Vigorous?" After taking into consideration things that might affect fertility, such as contraceptive use, smoking, and age, Dr. Rich-Edwards and her colleagues found that vigorous activity actually offered some protection against ovulatory infertility. Every hour of vigorous activity per week translated into a 7 percent reduction in risk, with the lowest risk of infertility among women who exercised vigorously for at least five hours a week.[9] The relation between vigorous activity and infertility was partly due to its strong connection with weight control. But even when weight was mathematically erased as an issue, vigorous activity was still beneficial.

Brisk walking and other moderate activities didn't improve fertility as vigorous activities did. But they didn't hurt, either.

Do these findings from the Nurses' Health Study contradict the work of Dr. Frisch and others? Not at all. Exercising too much in combination with being too lean can throw a monkey wrench into the delicate machinery of ovulation. But only a small fraction of American women are at the too lean end of the weight spectrum. The majority are closer to the other end. For them, an increase in exercise is a blessing, not a curse, for pregnancy and long-term health.

The take-home messages of Dr. Rich-Edwards's study are these:

- Exercise, including some vigorous exercise, should be on the to-do list of almost every woman who wants to get pregnant, especially those who are overweight.
- The vast majority of women need more exercise, not less.

Any type of activity is good for the body. Walking, vacuuming the floor, climbing stairs, dancing, lifting weights—they all keep the muscles, heart, lungs, and other body parts in shape. The more variety, the better, because exercise only affects the muscles that are being worked, and you reap the most benefit from working all your muscles. This is one reason why the Surgeon General and other experts routinely promote a variety of moderate physical activities as the path to good health. Another, perhaps more cynical, reason is that relatively few Americans heeded the earlier recommendations for vigorous activity three to five days a week.[4]

Make no mistake: walking and other moderate physical activities are good for you and are worlds better than doing nothing. But don't be afraid to turn up the intensity of your workouts. In just about every study of moderate activity, the researchers almost invariably acknowledge that they observed even greater benefits with vigorous activity.

That seems to be the case for fertility. For women who are overweight, gradually increasing the amount and intensity of daily physical activity is one route to improving the chances of having a baby. If your weight is in the healthy range or you are on the slim side, vigorous activity is still OK. Just don't overdo it. As a general guide, try to include vigorous activities like jogging or running, fast bicycling, aerobic dance, swimming, singles tennis, or cross-country skiing for about half of your exercise routine. That could mean doing a vigorous activity three times a week for half an hour or six times a week for fifteen minutes.

▶Moderate or Vigorous?

The distinction between moderate and vigorous activity is a bit shaky. What's moderate for one person might be vigorous for another. Activities are usually rated by how they affect the body and with a measure called metabolic equivalents, or METs. One MET is the amount of energy you use while reading a book or watching television. The harder your body works during an activity, the higher an activity's MET score.

Here's how the federal Centers for Disease Control and Prevention define the two:

Moderate-Intensity Physical Activities
- Cause a modest increase in breathing or heart rate
- Don't interfere with normal conversation
- Have a "perceived exertion" of 11 to 14 on the Borg scale (see Table 11.2 later in this chapter)
- Earn a rating of 3 to 6 METs
- Burn three and a half to seven calories per minute

Examples of moderate activities include:

Home activities. Walking to work or the store, walking the dog, other moderate or brisk walking, mowing the lawn with a power mower, general lawn and garden maintenance.

Exercise and leisure. Roller-skating, leisurely bicycling, aerobic dancing, water aerobics, yoga, weight training and bodybuilding, ballroom or line dancing.

Sports. Golf, softball and baseball, doubles tennis, downhill skiing, coaching children's or adults' sports.

Vigorous-Intensity Physical Activities
- Cause a substantial increase in breathing or heart rate
- Make conversation difficult
- Have a "perceived exertion" of 15 or greater on the Borg scale
- Earn a rating greater than 6 METs
- Burn more than seven calories per minute

Examples of vigorous activities include:

Home activities. Carrying groceries upstairs, moving heavy furniture, performing heavy carpentry work, stacking firewood, mowing the lawn with a nonmotorized push mower.

■ **Exercise and leisure.** Jogging or running, fast bicycling, wheeling your wheelchair, backpacking, karate, step aerobics, using a stair-climber or rowing machine at a fast pace, cross-country skiing.

■ **Sports.** Most competitive sports, including soccer, swimming field hockey or ice hockey, lacrosse, singles tennis, and racquetball.

▶Eggcellent Exercise

Working your muscles is good—not bad—for ovulation and conception. It's an integral part of losing or controlling weight and keeping blood sugar and insulin in check.

As we point out in Chapter 10, being overweight can delay or even derail pregnancy. Although experts aren't totally certain why this is so, hormonal disturbances are probably at the root of the problem. Body fat, also known as adipose tissue, generates a variety of hormones that influence appetite, activity, weight, and reproduction. Some of these hormones are needed to promote ovulation; too much of them can shut it down. Others have a damaging effect on ovulation.

Equally important, every episode of exercise—especially vigorous, muscle-strengthening exercise—makes your muscles react more efficiently to insulin's "open up for sugar" signal. If they already do this well, the effect is small but still worthwhile. If your muscles are succumbing to the creeping insensitivity to insulin that often occurs with excess weight, age, or inactivity, a single exercise session speeds the entry of blood sugar into muscle cells and improves their sensitivity to insulin. The net result is lower blood sugar and insulin in the bloodstream. That's why exercise is an integral part of controlling type 2 diabetes, a condition caused by muscles' resistance to insulin. The effect fades in a day or so, which is why people with this condition should exercise every day. Keeping insulin and blood sugar in check is important for fertility. When they spike higher than they should after a meal or snack and linger longer than they should in the bloodstream, they disrupt the finely tuned balance of hormones needed to mature an egg and release it at just the right moment.

The Fertility Zone for Activity

Much as we would like to offer a single, succinct prescription for conception-boosting exercise, as the Surgeon General did for exercise and general health, we can't. Some women need more exercise than others, for their weight or moods, and others are active just because they enjoy it. Some who need to be active aren't, while a small number of others may be too active.

Instead of focusing on an absolute number, try aiming for the fertility zone. This is a range of exercise that offers the biggest window of opportunity for fertility. Being in the fertility zone means you aren't overdoing or underdoing exercise.

For most women, this means getting at least thirty minutes of exercise every day. But if you are carrying more pounds than is considered healthy for your frame (i.e., a BMI above 25), you may need to exercise for an hour or more. If you are quite lean (i.e., your BMI is 19 or below), aim for the middle of the exercise window for a few months. (See Figure 11.1.)

Keep in mind that the fertility zone is an ideal, not an absolute. Hospital delivery rooms are full of women who rarely, or never, exercise. Not everyone is so lucky. If you are having trouble getting pregnant, then maybe the zone is the right place for you.

Whether you classify yourself as a couch potato or an exercise aficionado, your fertility zone should include four distinct types of physical activity:

- Aerobic exercise
- Strength training
- Stretching
- Activities of daily living

Like a well-oiled team, this quartet works together to control weight, guard against high blood sugar and insulin, and keep your muscles limber and ready for exercise. They are also natural stress relievers, something that almost everyone coping with or worrying about infertility can use. The sections that follow offer an overview of these four intertwined aspects of exercise along with tips for putting them into

Figure 11.1 **The Fertility Zone for Activity**

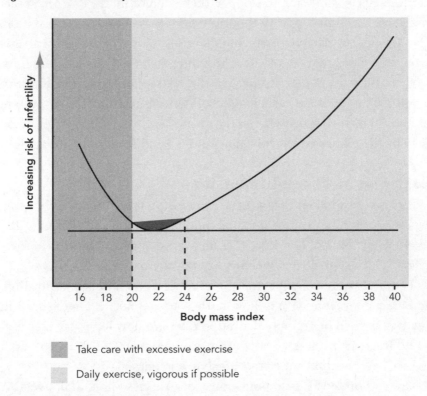

☐ Take care with excessive exercise

☐ Daily exercise, vigorous if possible

Physical activity, especially vigorous physical activity, can be a boon to *most* women trying to get pregnant. It's good for you if you weigh more than is ideal for your height (your BMI is above 25) or if your weight is in the healthy range (a BMI between 20–25). If you are relatively thin and lean, though, too much exercise or physical activity may interfere with ovulation.

play. For more detailed exercise plans, we recommend *The No Sweat Exercise Plan* by Harvey B. Simon, M.D.[10]

▶ Aerobic Exercise

Anything you do that makes your heart and lungs work substantially harder than they do while you are sitting qualifies as an aerobic activity. Think brisk walking, bicycling, cross-country skiing, jumping rope, swimming, aerobic dancing, and anything else that gets your blood circulating faster.

The term *aerobic* means "with oxygen." It was applied to exercise in the 1960s by Dr. Kenneth Cooper, then a major in the U.S. Air Force, based on his studies of fifty thousand servicemen and servicewomen. The twenty- to thirty-minute conditioning plans he outlined in his groundbreaking 1968 book, *Aerobics*, increase the body's demand for oxygen. Such workouts strengthen the heart and lungs and improve the flexibility of blood vessels. This allows the cardiovascular system to deliver oxygen more efficiently to the body. Aerobic activity also goes by the names cardiovascular exercise and endurance exercise.

Exercise in Three Dimensions

Aerobic exercise should be the centerpiece of your pregnancy-enhancing exercise program. Aim to do something aerobic on most days of the week. What? And for how long? The answers depend on the kind of exercise you choose to do and whether or not you are trying to lose weight.

Think of exercise as having three dimensions: intensity, duration, and frequency. Intensity is how hard you exercise. It's measured in calories burned per minute. Duration refers to how long you exercise, while frequency refers to how often. You can vary all three to find a type of exercise that suits your lifestyle and personality.

Say you prefer to keep your bouts of exercise short and sweet. A high-intensity activity such as tennis or vigorous cycling might be right for you. If intense isn't your thing, a less vigorous activity that you can do more often or for longer periods gives your body a similar workout.

Comparing brisk walking and working out on a rowing machine shows how this works. For a 155-pound person, thirty minutes of brisk walking would burn about 135 calories, while the same time on a rowing machine would burn about 420 calories. You can put this information to work another way: you can burn 300 calories with twenty-one minutes of rowing or sixty-seven minutes of brisk walking. Table 11.1 lists the intensities of fifteen aerobic exercises.

You also need to factor in weight control when planning how much to exercise. If one of your exercise goals is to lose a few pounds or to maintain your weight, thirty minutes a day may work if you're careful

Table 11.1 **Comparing Exercise Intensities**

The more intense an activity, the more calories it burns per minute. One measure of exercise intensity is the metabolic equivalent, or MET. The higher the MET, the more intense the activity.

Activity	METs	Minutes to Burn 300 Calories
Cross-country skiing, hard snow, uphill	16.5	15
Bicycle racing (over 20 mph)	16	16
Running, fast (10 mph)	16	16
Rowing machine, vigorous	12	21
In-line skating	12	21
Swimming, fast vigorous effort	10	26
Tennis, singles	8	32
Walking, fast (5 mph)	8	32
Slimnastics, Jazzercise	6	43
Mowing the lawn with a hand mower	6	43
Dancing, fast (disco, folk, square, line, Irish step, polka, contra, country)	4.5	57
Table tennis	4	64
Vacuuming	3.5	73
Walking, moderate speed (3 mph)	3.3	77
Croquet	2.5	102

These values are for a 155-pound person. Calories burned per minute would be smaller for a lighter person and larger for a heavier person.

about what and how much you eat. But you may need more—the Institute of Medicine says it can take sixty minutes or more of moderate-intensity activity a day to lose weight.[11] Here again, you can trade off duration for intensity. You can hit this goal with an hour of brisk walking or half an hour of jogging. You can also think of this as covering four miles, either walking or jogging.

Aerobic Options

Many exercise recommendations emphasize walking. And why not? It's free and easy, it doesn't require special training or equipment, and it can be done anytime and anywhere. Plus dozens of studies show that walking can prevent or help control high blood pressure, high cholesterol, heart disease, diabetes, peripheral artery disease, heart failure, and a host of other conditions. As a bonus, walking is a weight-bearing exercise that can help prevent osteoporosis.

If you are just starting, walk fast enough to get your heart pumping faster but not so fast that you have trouble talking. This corresponds to moderate exercise, as described in "How Hard Am I Working?" As your heart, lungs, and muscles get used to this pace, pick it up a bit. Aim for a brisk or fast pace (see "Step by Step").

Are you more interested in sports than walking? If so, tennis is a good option. In addition to being an aerobic sport that gives your heart and lungs a workout, it can be played at many different levels and well into old age.

If you'd rather get your exercise by working out on a machine, you'll burn the most calories on a treadmill. According to a comparison study from the Medical College of Wisconsin, you burn more calories with less perceived exertion (meaning you don't feel as though you are working as hard) with a treadmill; stair-steppers, rowing machines,

) HOW HARD AM I WORKING?

One of the easiest ways to measure how hard you are working is by using the Borg Scale of Perceived Exertion. (See Table 11.2.) It matches how hard you feel you are working with numbers from 6 to 20. The scale runs from "no feeling of exertion," which rates a 6, to "very, very hard," which rates a 19 or 20 and basically means you are exercising so hard you couldn't possibly push yourself any harder. Moderate activities usually clock in at 11 to 14 on the Borg scale, while vigorous activities usually rate a 15 or higher. Why does the scale run from 6 to 20 instead of 1 to 10? Its developer, Dr. Gunnar Borg, created it to roughly correspond to heart rates. Multiplying the Borg score by 10 gives you an approximate heart rate for a level of activity.

Table 11.2 **The Borg Scale**

Verbal Description of Your Exertion	Numeric Rating of Your Exertion	Examples
None	6	Reading this book, watching television
Very, very light	7 to 8	Tying your shoes
Very light	9 to 10	Chores that don't seem to take any effort, like washing the dishes
Fairly light	11 to 12	Walking through the grocery store or other activities that require effort but not enough to speed up your breathing
Somewhat hard	13 to 14	Brisk walking or other activities that require moderate effort and speed your heart and breathing but don't make you out of breath
Hard	15 to 16	Running, cross-country skiing, or other activities that take vigorous effort—your heart is pounding and breathing is very fast
Very hard	17 to 18	The highest level of activity you can sustain
Very, very hard	19 to 20	A finishing kick in a race or other burst of activity that you can't maintain for long

and cross-country trainers come next, all ahead of the standard stationary bicycle.[12]

Break It Up

A single long stretch of exercise a day works for some people. It is predictable and efficient. You warm up, stretch, work out, cool down, shower, and change just once. But what if you just can't fathom shoehorning thirty minutes of exercise into your day, let alone sixty? You don't need to do all your exercise at once. Breaking aerobic exercise into three or more ten-minute stints is just as good as doing it all at once.

STEP BY STEP

Want to know how fast you walk? You could have someone drive along-side you for a block or so and read off your pace from the car's speed-ometer. An easier way is to count how many steps you take in a minute. As long as you are walking on level ground, this general guide can gauge your pace:

- Slow = 80 steps per minute
- Moderate to brisk = 100 steps per minute
- Fast = 120 steps per minute
- Racewalking = more than 120 steps per minute

There's Strength in Resistance

Strength training, also called resistance training or weight training, builds and strengthens muscle. It does this by making the muscle resist an opposing force. This resistance causes a tiny bit of damage that the body repairs by building more muscle. The resistance can be supplied by your body's weight or by dumbbells, weighted cuffs, elastic bands, or special machines. No matter where the resistance comes from, put-ting a strain or load on your muscles makes them stronger.

Strength training is a fundamental part of fertility zone exercise because of its profound effect on blood sugar and insulin. It is a perfect natural medicine and works even better than most medications for con-trolling this potentially harmful duo. Strength training has many other benefits. The more muscle you have, the easier it is to control your weight, because muscle burns more calories than its equivalent in fat. When you work your muscles, they tug on the bones to which they are attached, and this builds bone, too. Strength training can make you look and feel better. It can improve your ability to carry out every-day activities, such as carrying groceries and climbing stairs. Stronger muscles mean better agility and balance, which translates into a lower risk of falling and injuring yourself.

There are two main types of resistance exercises: isotonic and iso-metric. During isotonic exercise, also called dynamic exercise, the muscle shortens and moves the attached joint. Raising a light weight from your knee to your shoulder or doing a push-up are examples of isotonic exercises. During isometric exercise, the muscle contracts but doesn't move the attached limb. Pushing your palms against each other or straining to lift an extremely heavy weight are examples of isometric exercise.

Isometric exercise is the quickest way to build muscle strength, but it can put unwanted stress on the heart and circulatory system. Isotonic exercise, on the other hand, builds muscle strength and endurance without excessively taxing your cardiovascular system. Lifting free weights or working out on the kind of weight or resistance machines in most gyms are all types of isotonic exercise.

If you are just embarking on a strength-training program, high-repetition, low-resistance exercises are the safest bet. You start out with a relatively light weight that you can lift at least eight times before the muscle gets fatigued; if you can do more than fifteen repetitions, increase the weight. As your muscles get stronger, increase the weight or the level of resistance every few sessions until you reach a sustainable plateau.

Unlike aerobic exercise, which should be done on most days, it's best to do strength training just two or three times a week. This gives your muscles a chance to recover fully between sessions.

Loosen Up

Stretching is another cornerstone of a safe, balanced exercise program. It won't do much for fertility, but it will do wonders for your muscles. Exercises that isolate and stretch the elastic fibers surrounding your muscles and tendons keep them limber. A well-stretched muscle moves more easily through its entire range of motion, resulting in better performance. The more limber you are, the easier it is to bend over and pick up a child or heft a sack of groceries. You'll stand taller, move more easily, and look better.

Until a few years ago, stretching before exercising was considered de rigueur for preventing sprains and other injuries. That practice fell out of favor after a few small trials showed it didn't offer much protection against muscle injuries. If you like to stretch before a workout, do it. But it's just as beneficial if you stretch after you've finished exercising or after a shower, before bed, or when you are stressed.

Gentle, gradual, yogalike stretches are best for most people. You assume a particular position, like standing with one foot on the floor and the other on a stair, then slowly use the weight of your body to stretch one set of muscles, tendons, and ligaments. The goal is to feel a mild pull on them. If it's painful, stop. When starting out, don't hold stretches for more than ten to fifteen seconds. As you become more limber, build up to twenty or thirty seconds.

Being aware of your breathing can help you stretch and relax at the same time. Start out by taking a deep breath, and then slowly let it out as you stretch. Visualize the body part you are stretching. After each stretch, relax your body, mind, and breathing. Wait for a short time (ten to thirty seconds) before repeating the stretch, and then move on to another part of your body.

You can stretch almost anywhere—at home, in the office, even while sitting in the car or on an airplane. Most stretches don't require any accessories, though a small towel can come in handy for a few. If you like instruction or group activities, yoga and Pilates classes are also excellent ways to get your ration of stretching.

▶Activity and Daily Life

Thirty minutes or so of purposeful exercise each day is great. It's even better if the rest of your day is punctuated—better yet, filled—with activity.

Grocery shopping, doing the laundry, pacing while you talk on the phone, walking or riding a bike to work, school, or shopping, even getting off the couch to change channels on the TV instead of using the remote—these activity bits can add up to make a big difference in the calories you burn each day (see "The Fidget Factor"). But don't let them take the place of exercise. Few daily activities give you the kind of sustained cardiovascular workout that exercise does.

Adding more activity bits to your day can be a challenge. Sometimes a little feedback can nudge you into action. Try wearing a pedometer for a few days. These descendants of the simple, pendulum-powered device that Leonardo da Vinci designed to count steps are inexpensive ($5 to $40) pager-sized devices. When clipped to a belt or pocket, a pedometer will clock every step you take, including those in the grocery store, running down to the basement to put in laundry, around the kitchen as you make dinner, and all the other steps you easily overlook. Using a pedometer for a week or so can help you get a handle on how active you are. Once you've figured out how many steps you take on an average day, try aiming for an extra thousand. Then aim higher.

Want more motivation? How about walking the equivalent of the Lewis and Clark Trail or the route of the famous Iditarod sled dog race without straying too far from home? A nonprofit organization called America on the Move sets you up with a virtual hike that you cover using steps recorded on a pedometer. The organization's website (www.americaonthemove.org) also offers tools for setting activity goals and tips for cutting back on calories.

▶The Fidget Factor

Staying on your feet when you can and moving, what Mayo Clinic endocrinologist James A. Levine calls nonexercise activity thermogenesis (NEAT), can help control weight and keep muscles healthy. Here's how Dr. Levine does it: when he's in his office, he walks at a slow but steady clip on the treadmill he uses instead of sitting in a chair. His computer, phone, and other office equipment are mounted above it so he can type, talk, even drink coffee while moving. Instead of meeting around a conference table, he and his colleagues talk while walking around a track. They believe that daily activity is so important that they have designed an Office of the Future that looks more like a gym than an office, with treadmills that serve as both desks and computer platforms and a two-lane walking track that functions as a meeting room. A desk-free Classroom of the Future that keeps kids active while they learn has also been tested in a public school in Rochester, Minnesota.

You don't have to add a treadmill to your office or in front of your TV (though that's not a bad idea) to add activity bits to your day. There are many things you can do in the privacy of your home or office or in the great outdoors that will work your muscles and burn extra calories.

- Whenever you can, use your feet or a bike to get yourself from one place to another.
- If you can't walk to work, take a five- or ten-minute walk before you hop in the car or before going into work. If you take public transportation, get off a stop or two early, if possible, and hoof it the rest of the way to work.
- When you drive to work or the store, instead of circling the parking lot waiting to pounce on the parking spot closest to the door, pull right into the one farthest away and then stroll to the entrance.
- At work, instead of printing to the printer on your desk, print to a communal one as far from your office as possible.
- On your lunch break, go window shopping instead of online shopping. If there's nothing of interest nearby, take a walk around your office building or parking lot.
- When talking on the phone, use a headset and pace instead of sitting.
- Take the stairs when you can, even if it's just for a few flights.
- Have a lawn? Try using an old-fashioned push mower instead of a power mower.

▶Topple Your Exercise Barriers

It's one thing to say, "Just do it." It's another to actually get moving. Cars, labor-saving devices, televisions, other machines and gadgets, and even the design and layout of our communities can subvert the need for muscle power and seduce us into sitting rather than moving.

Personal barriers also get in the way. These range from lack of time to worries that exercise will cause a heart attack or injury and limited access to safe places to exercise.

If you want to exercise but have trouble getting started or sticking with it, try taking the Barriers to Being Active quiz from the National Center for Chronic Disease Prevention and Health Promotion (available at www.cdc.gov/nccdphp/dnpa/physical/life). It can help you identify some of the things standing in your way.

Working several different activities into your day can help you meet your fitness goals and sidestep boredom. If you already have a structured exercise program in place, try supplementing it with recreation and daily activity. Or if you are active but don't exercise, try building a regular fitness program into your schedule—say, around a weekly tennis match or game of golf (no carts!). Table 11.3 suggests thirty different ways to burn calories.

You don't have to leap the barriers standing between you and a more active life in a single bound. Instead, try putting one foot in front of the other and walking around them.

Buddy Up

You probably turn to family members or friends all the time for help from everything to cleaning house to planning parties. Why not do the same thing for exercise?

Having an exercise buddy can help you—and you can help him or her—start or stick with exercise. Knowing that someone is waiting for you makes it tougher to skip a morning exercise class or an after-work run. On days when you are down, your buddy can pick you up, and vice versa. Having an exercise buddy can introduce a little friendly competition that can push each of you to higher limits. And for most people, exercising with someone else is more fun than going solo.

Try tapping your partner first. An Indiana University study found that couples who exercise together generally stick with it and are more active than those who go it alone.[13] If your partner already exercises, he or she can help you get in the groove. If not, your partner can certainly benefit as much as you will from exercise. Exercising together is also another way for both of you to work together toward an important goal.

Table 11.3 **Thirty Ways to Burn Calories**

You can burn calories hundreds of ways. Here are thirty examples, along with how many calories they burn in an hour. Some are things you can fit into your day as part of an active lifestyle. Others are sports and recreational activities you might do for pleasure, relaxation, or exercise.

Activity	METs*	Calories Burned in 60 Minutes		
		125-pound person	155-pound person	185-pound person
Conditioning Exercises				
Walking, brisk (3.5 mph)	3.8	216	268	320
Aerobics, low impact	5.0	284	352	420
Stationary cycling, low setting	5.0	284	352	420
Bicycling, leisurely (10–12 mph)	6.0	341	423	505
Swimming, leisurely	6.0	341	423	505
Ski machine, medium	9.0	511	634	757
Swimming, vigorous laps	10.0	568	705	841
Running (6 mph)	10.0	568	705	841
Bicycling, vigorous (14–16 mph)	10.0	568	705	841
Rowing machine, vigorous	12.0	682	845	1,009
Daily Activities				
Washing dishes	2.3	131	162	193
Food shopping with or without a cart	2.3	131	162	193
Cooking or preparing food	2.5	142	176	210
Walking slowly, putting away household items	3.0	170	211	252
Sweeping floors	3.3	188	233	278
Scrubbing floors	3.8	216	268	320
Playing with children, moderate active	4.0	227	282	336
General gardening	4.0	227	282	336
Raking the lawn	4.3	244	303	362
Carrying groceries upstairs	7.5	426	528	631

Sports, Leisure Activities				
Sexual activity (vigorous)	1.5	85	105	126
Hatha yoga, stretching	2.5	142	176	210
Ballroom dancing, slow (waltz, fox-trot, etc.)	3.0	170	211	252
Golf, using power cart	3.5	199	247	294
Tai chi	4.0	227	282	336
Golf, walking and carrying clubs	4.5	256	317	378
Cross-country skiing, slow or light effort	7.0	398	493	589
Racquetball, casual	7.0	398	493	589
Tennis, singles	8.0	455	564	673
Basketball, game	8.0	455	564	673

*METs stands for metabolic equivalents. One MET is the energy you use when sitting still. Heavier people burn more calories per minute than lighter people, so we have listed calories burned for three different representative weights.

Adapted from Ainsworth BE, Haskell WL, Whitt MC, Irwin ML, Swartz AM, Strath SJ, O'Brien WL, Bassett DR Jr, Schmitz KH, Emplaincourt PO, Jacobs DR Jr, and Leon AS. Compendium of physical activities: An update of activity codes and MET intensities. *Medicine and Science in Sports and Exercise* 2000; 32 (Suppl):S498–S516. You can see the complete list at http://prevention.sph.sc.edu/tools/compendium.htm.

If your partner won't budge, or prefers to exercise alone, see if you can enlist another family member, a friend, a neighbor, or a work colleague. The newest way to find an exercise buddy? You guessed it—the Internet. The online community craigslist (www.craigslist.org) is full of requests for exercise buddies, and there are even a handful of websites, like Exercise Friends (www.exercisefriends.com) and Find an Exercise Partner (www.findanexercisepartner.com), that can match you up with like-minded folks in your area. Local walking or running clubs are an even safer way to meet exercise partners.

Don't overlook your dog. Canine friends can make terrific exercise buddies. They're usually happy to go for a walk or run at any time and in any weather, which might give you the motivation you need to get out and exercise.

Of course, not everyone needs or wants companionship when she exercises. If you'd rather not have anyone see you exercise, get some exercise tapes or DVDs for a workout behind closed doors. Or maybe you prefer to greet the day in silence with a solitary morning run or wind down with a quiet session at the gym. Exercising by yourself is no worse, or no better, than working out with a companion. It's what it is, and if it works for you, keep it up.

Moving for Two

Exercise has gotten a bad rap when it comes to fertility. While the pioneering studies of Dr. Rose Frisch and her colleagues convincingly show that too much exercise coupled with too little stored energy can throw off or turn off ovulation in elite athletes, their work says nothing about the impact of usual exercise in normal-weight or overweight women. Common sense says that it can't be a big deterrent to conception. If it were, many of us wouldn't be here. Our ancestors worked hard to hunt, forage, clear and till fields, and travel from place to place. Early *Homo sapiens* burned twice as many calories each day as the average American does today and were fertile despite it—or because of it.[14]

Results from the Nurses' Health Study support this evolutionary perspective and show that exercise, particularly vigorous exercise, actually improves fertility. Exercising for at least thirty minutes on most days of the week (this would burn about two thousand calories a week) is a great place to start. It doesn't really matter how you exercise, as long as you find something other than your true love that moves you and gets your heart beating faster.

If you are already active and exercise most days of the week, congratulations. You are part of a rare—and healthy—group of women. Your exercise habit is good for your mood, your weight, your bones, your heart, and the rest of you. It will carry you through this stage of your life to middle age, menopause, and beyond. Before all that, it can help you get pregnant. If you aren't active and are trying to get pregnant, lace up your exercise shoes, load up your MP3 player, and belt out to your future child, "Baby, we were born to run."

· · · · · · · ·

Chapter 12

Putting It All Together

W e hope we have convinced you by now that a few changes in diet, weight, and activity can ignite ovulation and help you get pregnant faster and with fewer worries. These changes include:

- More slow carbs, fewer highly processed ones.
- More healthful unsaturated fats, no trans fat.
- More protein from plants, less from red meat.
- A serving or two a day of whole milk or other full-fat dairy foods, less skim milk and low-fat dairy foods.
- A daily multivitamin that contains at least 400 mcg of folic acid and 40 to 80 mg of iron.
- Coffee, tea, and alcohol in moderation, if at all, but no sugared sodas.
- Moving toward the fertility zone for weight (a body mass index between 20 and 24) and physical activity (thirty to sixty minutes a day, and don't be afraid of vigorous exercise).

While reading the previous chapters, you may have been silently tallying the overall effect of the Fertility Diet. Adding all of the reductions in risk gives an astonishing 300 percent reduction in ovulatory infertility—almost a guarantee for pregnancy!

Unfortunately, it doesn't work that way. The body functions much as ecologist Barry Commoner once said the environment does: everything is connected to everything else. How much and what kinds of carbohydrate you eat affect your fat and protein intake. Protein intake partly determines the fats you take in. Fruit and vegetable consumption affect all of these. Your daily activity level influences your weight, and vice versa, and both shape how much you eat.

Whenever we analyzed a different element of the Fertility Diet, we used statistical techniques to take into consideration the effects of all the other parts. These calculations gave us a way to keep everything else steady so we could see the impact of the one factor we were looking at. In our analysis of plant protein, for example, we adjusted for contributions to ovulatory infertility made by total calories, age, body mass index, smoking history, physical activity, use of multivitamins, and intake of iron and different types of fat.

What's more, several components of our plan may involve the same pathways: minimizing spikes in blood sugar and insulin, improving the sensitivity of tissues to insulin's "open up for sugar" signals, maintaining a fertility-boosting balance of female to male hormones, calming inflammation, and promoting the healthy development and release of a mature egg each month.

Like you, we wondered what would happen when you combine two, three, four, or more of the steps of the Fertility Diet. To answer that question, we devised a Fertility Diet score for every woman in the study. For each component of the Fertility Diet, we created a five-point scale. A woman got five points if she was in the group with the lowest risk of infertility, one point if she was in the highest risk group, and intermediate points for intermediate risks. For example, a woman in the highest category of daily vegetable protein intake would get five points because greater intake of vegetable protein is associated with protection against ovulatory infertility, while a woman in the highest category of low-fat dairy intake would get one point because low-fat dairy is associated with an increased risk. We did this for glycemic load, the ratio of monounsaturated to trans fats, vegetable protein, animal protein, full-fat dairy, low-fat dairy, multivitamin use, and iron intake. We added the points to create each woman's Fertility Diet score.

Women in the top fifth of the scores were 66 percent less likely to have had trouble with ovulatory infertility than women with the lowest scores. In general, the women with the highest scores had adopted three or four of the recommendations suggested in this book.[1] Infertility from other causes was also reduced. We checked to see if following the Fertility Diet worked better for some groups of women. It did. Among women over age thirty-five, those with the highest Fertility Diet scores were 72 percent less likely to have experienced ovulatory infertility. Among women who were in the fertility zone for weight, those with the highest scores were 74 percent less likely to have experienced ovulatory infertility.

We also tested the effectiveness of the Fertility Diet another way, by comparing rates of ovulatory infertility with the number of Fertility Diet habits the nurses followed. This time we included weight (as body mass index) and exercise along with the list of dietary changes used for the Fertility Diet score. As shown in Figure 12.1, compared to women who didn't follow any of the habits, those who followed one of them had a 30 percent lower risk of ovulatory infertility. Each additional strategy further reduced the chance of experiencing ovulating infertility. Put another way, compared to women who followed five or more Fertility Diet habits, those who didn't follow any were six times more likely to have experienced ovulatory infertility.

We couldn't determine the effect of following six, seven, or even all ten of the steps, because only a few of the participants followed five or more of them. But it is likely that the more elements of the fertility plan you follow, the more protection you gain against ovulation-related infertility.

Will following all ten steps guarantee that you will get pregnant quickly or at all? Unfortunately, no. Our ten-step plan can help improve ovulation in several different ways. And in a large group of women, the elements of the Fertility Diet alone and together substantially reduced the chances of experiencing ovulatory infertility. "Substantially reduced" is great, but it doesn't mean complete prevention or a guarantee of pregnancy.

Figure 12.1 **Additive Benefits**

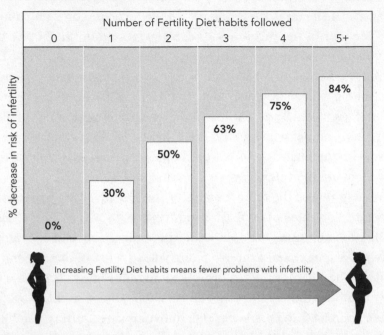

Following one of the Fertility Diet's strategies is helpful; adding others is even better. Compared to women in the Nurses' Health Study who didn't follow any of the strategies, those who followed one were 30 percent less likely to have encountered ovulatory infertility. Each addition further lowered the risk, down to a substantial 84 percent reduction among women who followed five or more of the strategies.

▶Start Strong and Improvise

A piano playing a jazzy standard like "Melancholy Baby" emanates a lovely sound. Adding a vibraphone brings depth and unexpected harmonies. Kick in a bass, a saxophone or two, and some drums, and you have the vibrant, responsive sound of a jazz band. The Fertility Diet is a bit like this. Following one of the steps is helpful. Adopting two, three, four, or more gives you even more protection and greater flexibility.

Jumping from a "regular" diet to the Fertility Diet all at once is a tall order. A smart option is to start with the essentials and work your way up from there. Where to start? We think these steps are vital for everyone:

- Take a multivitamin-multimineral with at least 400 micrograms (mcg) of folic acid and 40 milligrams (mg) of iron every day.
- Lose weight if needed.
- Exercise.
- Avoid trans fats.
- Don't smoke.

Taking a daily multivitamin-multimineral supplement improves fertility and ensures that you have enough folic acid in your system when you get pregnant. This vitamin is also needed to prevent birth defects such as spina bifida. Losing weight, if needed, and exercising are two of the best ways to improve your body's sensitivity to insulin. This will smooth out the blood sugar and insulin roller coaster, an essential step for improving fertility. Avoiding trans fats improves insulin sensitivity, too, and also cools inflammation throughout the body. This dual effect can foster ovulation and conception and promotes healthy development in a new and rapidly growing embryo. Avoiding cigarette smoke, yours or someone else's, can also improve fertility. Although we didn't explore the effect of smoking on fertility in the Nurses' Health Study (there were too few smokers for the results to be meaningful), solid research has established that women who smoke take longer to get pregnant on their own or with assisted reproduction, are more likely to be diagnosed with infertility, and are more likely to miscarry than nonsmokers.

What to do next? That's up to you. Pick a piece of the Fertility Diet that appeals to you or one you think would be easy to put into practice. If you are partial to carbohydrates, try out some new whole grains, replace your usual pasta with a whole-grain variety, and cut back on refined starches and potatoes. Maybe you have been hankering to tone down your reliance on carbohydrates and eat more protein. Now is a good time to do that—just be sure to put plant protein to work for you. Add more beans and nuts as well as eggs and fish; let red meat be a treat instead of your daily fare. This is also a great time to get over your fear of fats. Add healthful, ovulation-enhancing unsaturated fats to your diet by using olive oil, canola oil, and other vegetable oils in place of butter or hard margarine and by eating nuts. Swapping red meat for fish rich in omega-3 fats can boost fertility; these healthful fats are also important for your baby's development. If you enjoy milk and other dairy products but have been consuming mostly skim milk or low-fat dairy foods, try having a glass of whole milk, full-fat yogurt, or a piece of rich cheese each day. (Some of the recipes in Chapter 13 offer new ways to add whole milk or full-fat cheeses to your diet.) If dairy foods aren't your thing, skip them. There are plenty of other things you can do to improve your fertility.

▶Have It Your Way

The fertility plan we recommend isn't governed by strict rules. Like jazz, it is open to experimentation and improvisation. Each part of the plan can stand on its own. But doing the parts together brings harmony to the diverse processes leading to ovulation and conception and so increases your chances of getting pregnant. It also puts you on the road to healthy habits that are good for a pregnancy, for a developing baby, and for a lifetime of good health.

SEND US YOUR FEEDBACK

If you try the Fertility Diet, we would love to hear about the changes you made, how you accomplished them, and if they worked for you. You can leave comments at www.thefertilitydiet.com, send a message to mail@thefertilitydiet.com, or drop us a line at The Fertility Diet, c/o Harvard Health Publications, 10 Shattuck Street, 2nd Floor, Boston, MA 02115.

Chapter 13

Meal Plans and Recipes

T heory is one thing; real life is another. It's easy to say, "Include more full-fat milk or dairy products," "Get more iron from plants," or "Choose slow carbs instead of highly processed ones." Putting such recommendations into practice, though, takes the kind of thought and planning you don't always have at the beginning or end of a busy day. To give you a head start, we asked Maureen Callahan, a Denver-based dietitian par excellence, to create a week's worth of meal plans and fifteen delicious recipes that offer ideas for putting the book's recommendations into practice.

The meal plans and recipes don't contain any artificial trans fats. Fish, eggs, beans, nuts, and whole milk or full-fat dairy products, rather than red meat, provide the protein. Even though the daily meal plans include full-fat dairy foods, they still keep saturated fat levels in check. There are plenty of fruits and vegetables, slow carbs, and healthful unsaturated fats.

Notice that this isn't a diet of deprivation. Instead, it is drawn from the bountiful cornucopia of foods available in most supermarkets. And it is meant to satisfy your appetite, not merely keep it at bay.

Each day's menu averages out to around two thousand calories, the amount that health experts say the typical healthy young woman needs to stay fit. Depending on your size and activity level, this could be just right, too much, or not quite enough. But it is a good starting point and gives you examples that can guide you to the adaptations that are right for your journey to pregnancy.

In the meal plans that follow, *italics* identify entries for which recipes are provided.

Monday

■ **BREAKFAST**
Cooked oatmeal (1 cup)
Toasted slivered almonds (¼ cup)
Blueberries (1 cup)
Whole milk (1 cup)

■ **LUNCH**
Grilled Salmon Sushi
Sliced cucumbers (1 cup) with rice vinegar
Bartlett pear
Tea

■ **AFTERNOON SNACK**
Hard-boiled egg
Roasted red pepper or plain hummus (¼ cup)
Carrot or celery sticks (10–20)

■ **SUPPER**
Broccoli and White Bean Gratin or *Baked Cauliflower with Four Cheeses*
Field greens (2 cups) with cherry tomatoes (½ cup), olive oil (2 teaspoons), and a splash of vinegar
Sliced strawberries (1 cup)

■ **EVENING SNACK**
1 tablespoon peanut butter
1 apple, sliced

Tuesday

■ **BREAKFAST**
Whole wheat toast (1 slice)
Almond butter (1 tablespoon)

Vanilla soy milk yogurt (1 cup)

Sliced peaches (1 cup)

Coffee or tea

■ **LUNCH**

Black bean salad: black beans (⅓ cup), scallions and red peppers
(2 tablespoons each), olive oil (2 teaspoons), splash of vinegar

Curried Pumpkin Soup (1½ cups)

Fresh cantaloupe (½ melon)

Sparkling water

■ **AFTERNOON SNACK**

Mixed nuts (1 ounce)

■ **SUPPER**

Asian Salmon Burger

Steamed bok choy (1½ cups) with lemon olive oil (2 teaspoons)

Brown basmati rice (¾ cup)

Fresh sliced mango and pineapple (1 cup)

■ **EVENING SNACK**

Fresh grapes (1½ cups)

Havarti cheese with dill (½ ounce)

Wednesday

■ **BREAKFAST**

Banana-walnut smoothie: whole-milk vanilla yogurt (1 cup) blended
with frozen banana slices (1 cup), honey (1 teaspoon), toasted
chopped walnuts (1 tablespoon), dash of nutmeg, and crushed
ice (½ cup)

Rye crackers, crispbread style (2)

Cheddar cheese cubes (½ ounce)

■ **LUNCH**

Three-bean salad (2 cups)

Avocado (½ small)

Tangerines (2)

■ **AFTERNOON SNACK**

4 dried apricot halves

1 ounce shelled pistachio nuts

■ **SUPPER**

Orange-Glazed Salmon

Steamed napa cabbage (1½ cups) with olive oil (2 teaspoons)

Baked sweet potato (1 small)

Blueberries and raspberries (1 cup)

■ **EVENING SNACK**

Macintosh apple

Thursday

■ **BREAKFAST**

Scrambled eggs (2) with chopped chilies cooked in canola oil
    (1 teaspoon)

Fresh tomato salsa (½ cup)

Avocado (¼ whole)

Corn tortilla (2)

Fresh pineapple chunks (1 cup)

■ **LUNCH**

Red Lentil, Toasted Almond, and Ginger Soup

Chopped romaine lettuce (2 cups) with sliced red onion (¼ cup)
    and olive oil (1 tablespoon)

Carrot sticks (1 cup)

■ **AFTERNOON SNACK**

Roasted peanuts (¼ cup)

Raisins (2 tablespoons)

■ **SUPPER**

Grilled Moroccan Tuna

Steamed broccoli (1 cup)

Brown rice blend (½ cup)

Olive oil (2 teaspoons)

Sliced kiwifruit and strawberries (1 cup)

■ **EVENING SNACK**
Bartlett pear
Gorgonzola cheese (½ ounce)

Friday

■ **BREAKFAST**
Bran flakes with raisins (1½ cups)
Pecan halves (3 tablespoons)
Soy milk (1 cup)
Red grapefruit (1 whole)

■ **LUNCH**
Baby spinach leaves (2 cups)
Walnut oil (1 tablespoon) and fresh figs (2)
Creamy Parsnip–Carrot Soup

■ **AFTERNOON SNACK**
Fresh apricots (2)
Roasted almonds (1 ounce)

■ **SUPPER**
Grilled mahi mahi (6 ounces)
Whole-grain garlic couscous (1 cup)
Sesame Green Beans
Tangerine

■ **EVENING SNACK**
Cinnamon baked apple
Toasted chopped walnuts (1 tablespoon)

Saturday

■ **BREAKFAST**
Whole wheat English muffin
Peanut butter (1 tablespoon)
Low-sugar orange marmalade (1 tablespoon)
Whole-milk lemon yogurt (1 cup)
Blackberries and chopped kiwifruit (1 cup)

■ LUNCH
Spinach-mushroom salad (2 cups) with olive oil (1 tablespoon)
Black Olive Pilaf with Roasted Vegetables
Whole-grain baguette (1-ounce slice)
Fresh cantaloupe and strawberries (1½ cups)

■ AFTERNOON SNACK
Bell pepper strips (1 cup)
Hummus (¼ cup)
Pistachio nuts (¼ cup)

■ SUPPER
Mixed greens (2 cups) with balsamic vinegar and olive oil
    (1 tablespoon)
Chili-Spiced Shrimp
Mashed acorn squash (½ cup)
Roasted asparagus (1 cup)
Chopped fresh papaya and mango (1 cup)

■ EVENING SNACK
Dark chocolate (1 ounce)
Dried blueberries (⅓ cup)

Sunday

■ BREAKFAST
Fresh Corn and Cheddar Soufflé
Whole-grain toast (1 slice)
Blackberry jam (1 tablespoon)
Seasonal fresh fruit salad (1½ cups)

■ LUNCH
Guacamole (⅓ cup)
Poblano and Black Bean Chili
Red or green grapes (1 cup)

■ AFTERNOON SNACK
Carrot sticks (1 cup)
Fresh tomato salsa (½ cup)

■ SUPPER

Mesclun mix (2 cups) with olive oil (2 teaspoons)

Pecan-Crusted Tilapia with Mango Salsa

Steamed yellow squash with crushed red pepper flakes (1½ cups)

Bulgur (½ cup)

Fresh orange sections with mint (1 cup)

■ EVENING SNACK

Chocolate or coffee whole-milk yogurt (½ cup)

Slivered almonds (2 tablespoons)

■ DAILY AVERAGE FOR THE WEEK

Calories: 1,999; protein: 86 g; fiber: 47 g; sodium: 1,742 mg; saturated fat: 17 g

Creamy Parsnip–Carrot Soup

With 90 mcg per cup, parsnips are a rich source of folate. Combining them with carrots, celery, and a bit of potato tames the sweetness of this root vegetable and makes for a thick savory soup. Each main dish serving of soup contains one cup of whole milk.

1 1-ounce slice whole-grain bread

1 tablespoon olive oil, divided

3 cloves garlic, minced

1 cup chopped onion

1 cup chopped celery

½ teaspoon salt, divided

1½ cups peeled, chopped parsnips (about 4 ounces)

1 cup peeled, diced carrot

½ cup peeled, chopped potato

4 cups whole milk

½ cup vegetable broth

¼ teaspoon freshly ground pepper

¼ cup chopped fresh parsley

1½ tablespoons fresh thyme leaves

¾ teaspoon finely grated lemon zest

2 tablespoons lemon juice

2 tablespoons pine nuts, toasted

1. Place the bread in a minichopper or blender and pulse until the bread becomes evenly crumbly. Set the bread crumbs aside.

2. Heat 2 teaspoons of the olive oil in a Dutch oven or large saucepan over medium heat. Add half of the garlic and cook 1 minute. Stir in the bread crumbs and continue to cook 2 to 3 minutes, or until the bread crumbs are toasted. Remove the bread crumbs to a plate.

3. Wipe the pan with a paper towel and add the remaining 1 teaspoon of oil. Add the onion and celery and sauté over medium heat for 5 to 6 minutes, or until the vegetables are tender. Stir in the remaining

garlic and ¼ teaspoon salt; cook 30 seconds. Add the parsnips, carrots, potato, milk, and broth and bring to a boil. Reduce heat and simmer for 24 to 28 minutes, or until vegetables are tender. Stir in the pepper and remaining ¼ teaspoon salt and cook 1 minute.

4. Place the hot soup, parsley, and thyme in a blender; blend, with the lid partially open so that steam can escape, until pureed. Return to the pot to keep warm. Just before serving, stir in lemon zest and lemon juice. Spoon soup into bowls, garnish with pine nuts and bread crumbs, and serve.

Yield: 4 1½-cup servings

Calories: 333; protein: 12 g; carbohydrate: 39 g; fiber: 5 g; sodium: 564 mg; fat: 16 g (saturated: 6.4 g; monounsaturated: 6.1 g; polyunsaturated: 2.3 g; trans: 0.3 g); cholesterol: 34 mg; folate: 82 mcg; iron: 2 mg

Red Lentil, Toasted Almond, and Ginger Soup

Lentils are a good source of both folate and iron. The red ones lend an attractive color to this soup, but green or brown lentils will work just as well. If you've already used your one-cup allowance of whole milk for the day, substitute vegetable broth or nondairy milks (soy, rice, or almond) for the whole milk.

    2 teaspoons canola oil
    1½ cups chopped onions
    3 cloves garlic, minced
    2½ teaspoons freshly grated ginger
    2½ teaspoons garam masala (Indian spice blend)
    1 teaspoon ground coriander
    ¾ teaspoon salt, divided
    ⅛ teaspoon cayenne pepper
    4 cups whole milk
    1 cup red lentils
    ¼ cup slivered almonds, toasted
    ½ cup plain almond milk (such as Almond Breeze)
    ½ teaspoon freshly ground black pepper
    Chopped fresh cilantro (optional)

1. Heat the oil in a Dutch oven or large saucepan over medium heat. Add the onions and cook 3 to 5 minutes, or until tender. Stir in the garlic and ginger and cook 2 minutes. Add the garam masala, the coriander, ¼ teaspoon of the salt, and the cayenne and cook 1 minute. Add the milk and lentils and bring to a boil; reduce heat and simmer 14 to 18 minutes, or until the lentils are tender.

2. Place the lentil mixture and almonds in a blender, with the lid slightly ajar so that steam can escape, and puree until smooth. Return the soup to the pan. Stir in the almond milk, remaining ½ teaspoon of salt, and pepper; cook for 1 minute.

3. Spoon the soup into shallow bowls; garnish with cilantro, if desired.

Yield: 4 1½-cup servings

Calories: 416; protein: 22 g; carbohydrate: 48 g; fiber: 9 g; sodium: 600 mg; fat: 16 g (saturated: 6.1 g; monounsaturated: 6.9 g; polyunsaturated: 2 g; trans: 0.3 g); cholesterol: 34 mg; folate: 27 mcg; iron: 3 mg

Curried Pumpkin Soup

This quick soup takes less than thirty minutes to prepare and comes together with ingredients that are probably already in your pantry. Pair it with a vegetable-rich salad and a whole-grain roll.

    2 tablespoons olive oil
    1½ cups chopped onion
    ½ cup diced carrot
    ¾ teaspoon salt, divided
    2 teaspoons curry powder
    1 teaspoon mustard seed
    1 teaspoon turmeric
    ½ teaspoon ground coriander
    ⅛ to ¼ teaspoon cayenne pepper
    4 cups whole milk
    ½ cup vegetable broth
    1 15-ounce can pumpkin
    ⅓ cup chopped fresh cilantro
    ¼ teaspoon freshly ground black pepper

1. Heat the oil in a Dutch oven or large saucepan over medium heat. Add the onions and carrots and cook 6 to 8 minutes, stirring frequently, or until vegetables are tender. Stir in ½ teaspoon of the salt and the curry powder, mustard seed, turmeric, coriander, and cayenne; cook 2 minutes to toast the spices. Add the milk, broth, and pumpkin and bring to a boil; reduce heat and simmer for 10 minutes.

2. Place the soup in a blender and puree, with the lid ajar so that steam can escape, until smooth. Return the soup to the pan; stir in the cilantro, remaining ¼ teaspoon of salt, and pepper. Keep warm until ready to serve.

Yield: 6 1½-cup servings

Calories: 297; protein: 10 g; carbohydrate: 30 g; fiber: 5 g; sodium: 640 mg; fat: 17 g (saturated: 6.7 g; monounsaturated: 7.9 g; polyunsaturated; 1.1 g; trans: 0.3 g); cholesterol: 34 mg; folate: 43 mcg; iron: 3 mg

Broccoli and White Bean Gratin

Cannellini beans are a good source of both iron and folate; broccoli also has small amounts of folate. Frozen broccoli florets are a quick substitute; just follow package directions for cooking and then proceed with the recipe. Keep in mind that each serving offers one-half cup of whole milk and one-half ounce of full-fat cheese.

  1½ pounds broccoli tops
  1½ tablespoons olive oil, divided
  ½ cup finely chopped onion
  3 cups whole milk, divided
  2 tablespoons chopped fresh thyme
  1 clove garlic, minced
  ⅛ teaspoon nutmeg
  ¼ cup all-purpose flour
  ⅔ cup freshly grated Parmesan cheese, divided
  ¼ teaspoon freshly ground black pepper
  ½ teaspoon salt, divided
  2 15-ounce cans cannellini beans, rinsed and drained
  2 1-ounce slices whole wheat bread

1. Preheat the oven to 400°F.

2. Trim the broccoli into florets and cut the stalks into small pieces. Bring water to a boil in a Dutch oven. Add the broccoli, cover, and steam for 4 minutes. Drain well and set aside.

3. Add ½ tablespoon of the oil to the Dutch oven and heat over medium heat. Stir in the onions and sauté 2 to 3 minutes. Add 2½ cups of the milk, the thyme, the garlic, and the nutmeg and reduce heat to low; let the mixture steep for 10 minutes.

4. Place the remaining ½ cup of the milk in a small bowl; whisk in the flour. Whisk the flour-milk mixture into a pan with the remaining milk mixture and cook over medium heat until thick, stirring occa-

sionally at first and then frequently as the mixture thickens. This will take about 6 to 8 minutes. Remove from heat and stir in half of the Parmesan, the pepper, and ¼ teaspoon of the salt.

5. Combine the beans and cooked broccoli with the remaining ¼ teaspoon of salt in a small bowl. Let stand 2 minutes. Add the bean mixture to a pot and stir gently to mix. Place the bean-broccoli mixture into a 9″ × 13″ shallow baking dish coated with ½ teaspoon of the olive oil.

6. Place the bread in a minichopper or blender and pulse until bread crumbs form. Combine the bread crumbs, remaining Parmesan, and remaining 2½ teaspoons of oil; sprinkle evenly over the bean mixture. Bake at 400°F for 20 minutes, or until bubbly.

Yield: 6 1-cup servings

Calories: 337; protein: 18 g; carbohydrate: 42 g; fiber: 10 g; sodium: 591 mg; fat: 12 g (saturated: 5 g; monounsaturated: 4.7 g; polyunsaturated: 1.5 g; trans: 0.1 g); cholesterol: 25 mg; folate: 105 mcg; iron: 4 mg

Baked Cauliflower with Four Cheeses

Frozen cauliflower florets can be easily substituted for the fresh cauliflower. Cook them according to package directions and then proceed with the recipe. Each serving contains three-quarters of a cup of milk and about one-half ounce of cheese.

¼ teaspoon salt, divided
1 head of cauliflower (about 2½ pounds), trimmed and broken into florets
¼ cup all-purpose flour
3 cups whole milk, divided
2 tablespoons shredded fontina cheese (about ½ ounce)
2 tablespoons crumbled Gorgonzola cheese (about ½ ounce)
2 tablespoons shredded mozzarella (about ½ ounce)
1 tablespoon freshly grated Parmesan cheese (about ¼ ounce)
⅜ teaspoon freshly ground black pepper
1 tablespoon olive oil, divided
2 1-ounce slices whole-grain bread, torn into pieces

1. Preheat the oven to 400°F.

2. Bring 4 quarts of water to a boil in a large Dutch oven or stockpot. Add ⅛ teaspoon of the salt and the cauliflower. Cover and cook 3 minutes, or until crisp-tender. Drain the cauliflower and set aside.

3. Place the flour in a saucepan. Stir in ½ cup of the milk and whisk until smooth. Place the pan over medium heat and gradually add the remaining milk. Cook, whisking frequently, until the mixture begins to thicken, about 6 to 7 minutes. Remove from heat and stir in cheeses, the remaining ⅛ teaspoon salt, and pepper. Stir in the cauliflower. Lightly coat an 11″ × 7″ baking dish with ½ teaspoon of the olive oil; spread the cauliflower mixture evenly into it.

4. Place the bread in a minichopper or blender and pulse until ground into bread crumbs. Combine the bread crumbs and remaining 2½ teaspoons of olive oil and sprinkle the mixture evenly over the cauliflower mixture. Bake at 400°F for 15 minutes, or until bubbly. Let stand 5 minutes before serving.

Yield: 4 1½-cup servings

Calories: 291; protein: 14 g; carbohydrate: 27 g; fiber: 4 g; sodium: 498 mg; fat: 15 g (saturated: 7.3 g; monounsaturated: 5.5 g; polyunsaturated: 1 g; trans: 0 g); cholesterol: 39 mg; folate: 94 mcg; iron: 2 mg

Fresh Corn and Cheddar Soufflé

Serve this soufflé for breakfast or as a light supper. Any leftovers can be easily reheated for another meal. Just keep in mind that each serving delivers a half-cup serving of whole milk and a half-ounce of full-fat cheese.

1 ½ teaspoons olive oil, divided

½ cup chopped red onion

½ teaspoon salt, divided

3 cups fresh white sweet corn kernels (about 4 ears)

2 cups whole milk

4 large eggs, yolks and whites separated

2 tablespoons whole-grain cornmeal

2 tablespoons all-purpose flour

¼ teaspoon freshly ground black pepper

½ teaspoon cream of tartar

2 ounces extra sharp shredded cheddar cheese

¼ cup finely chopped fresh basil or thyme

1 tablespoon oil-packed sun-dried tomato pieces, drained and finely chopped

1. Preheat the oven to 375°F.

2. Heat a nonstick skillet over medium heat; add ½ teaspoon of the oil and heat. Add the onions and sauté for 2 to 3 minutes, or until tender. Stir in ¼ teaspoon of the salt. Remove from heat.

3. Place 1 cup of the corn in a blender or food processor; process until pureed. Stir the pureed corn into the onion mixture along with the milk, egg yolks, cornmeal, flour, remaining ¼ teaspoon salt, and pepper.

4. Place the egg whites in a bowl; add the cream of tartar and beat with a mixer at high speed, until stiff peaks form. Carefully stir one-third of the egg white mixture into the corn mixture. Fold in

the remaining egg white mixture, cheese, basil or thyme, and sun-dried tomatoes. Coat an 11″ × 7″ baking dish with the remaining 1 teaspoon of oil and spoon in the mixture. Bake at 375°F for 35 to 40 minutes, or until puffy and set.

5. Cut into 8 squares and serve.

Yield: 4 2-square servings

Calories: 287; protein: 15 g; carbohydrate: 31 g; fiber: 4 g; sodium: 477 mg; fat: 13 g (saturated: 5 g; monounsaturated: 5.1 g; polyunsaturated: 1.8 g; trans: 0 g); cholesterol: 226 mg; folate: 93 mcg; iron: 2 mg

Sesame Green Beans

This side dish can be served hot or cold. The green beans are a good source of folate, and the sesame seeds (which you can sometimes find already toasted) also contain a little bit of folate.

> 1 pound green beans, trimmed
> 1 teaspoon canola oil
> 1 teaspoon toasted sesame oil
> 1 tablespoon toasted sesame seeds
> 1 teaspoon soy sauce
> ¼ teaspoon salt
> ¼ teaspoon freshly ground black pepper

1. Steam the green beans over boiling water 4 minutes. Place in a colander and rinse with cold water. Drain well.

2. Place a large nonstick skillet over medium heat. Add the canola and sesame oils and heat over medium high heat. Add the beans and stir-fry 1 to 2 minutes, or until the beans are crisp-tender. Remove from heat and toss with the sesame seeds, soy sauce, salt, and pepper.

Yield: 4 4-ounce servings

Calories: 64; protein: 2 g; carbohydrate: 8 g; fiber: 4 g; sodium: 231 mg; fat: 4 g (saturated: 0.4 g; monounsaturated: 1.5 g; polyunsaturated: 1.3 g; trans: 0 g); cholesterol: 0 mg; folate: 39 mcg; iron: 1.3 mg

Grilled Moroccan Tuna

Because fresh tuna is higher in mercury than many other fish, the Food and Drug Administration recommends eating no more than six ounces per week. If you're concerned about even that amount, substitute a low-mercury fish, like salmon or tilapia, for the tuna.

1 teaspoon paprika

1 teaspoon sugar

½ teaspoon kosher or coarse salt

½ teaspoon ground ginger

½ teaspoon coriander

½ teaspoon allspice

½ teaspoon black pepper

¼ teaspoon ground mustard

¼ teaspoon cumin

4 6-ounce yellowfin tuna steaks, about 1 inch thick

2 teaspoons olive or canola oil

1. Combine the paprika, sugar, salt, ginger, coriander, allspice, pepper, mustard, and cumin in a shallow bowl.

2. Prepare the grill or an indoor grill pan.

3. Dredge the tuna steaks in the spice mixture, coating well on both sides. Drizzle the oil evenly over the tuna and place on the grill; cook 2 to 3 minutes on each side, or until desired degree of doneness.

Yield: 4 1-fillet servings

Calories: 213; protein: 40 g; carbohydrate: 2 g; fiber: 1 g; sodium: 299 mg; fat: 4 g (saturated: 0.7 g; monounsaturated: 1.9 g; polyunsaturated: 0.8 g; trans: 0 g); cholesterol: 77 mg; folate: 4 mcg; iron: 2 mg

Grilled Salmon Sushi

If you are a sushi fan, you'll know that brown rice isn't the authentic rice that sushi chefs use. But short-grain brown rice is plenty sticky for sushi and also delivers a healthy amount of fiber. The flat tail end of a salmon fillet works best here because it allows for thin slices that are easy to roll into sushi. Serve sushi with the traditional condiments of soy sauce, pickled ginger, and wasabi.

2 cups uncooked short-grain brown rice (such as Lundberg)
6 tablespoons seasoned rice vinegar
1 8-ounce tail end skinless, boneless salmon fillet, about ½-inch thick
⅛ teaspoon salt
6 nori (seaweed) sheets
12 thin stalks asparagus, trimmed and steamed
1 avocado, peeled and thinly sliced
½ red bell pepper, thinly sliced
1 tablespoon wasabi (Japanese horseradish)

1. Prepare the rice according to the package directions without salt or fat. Stir in the vinegar; cover and cool to room temperature.

2. Prepare the grill or an indoor grill pan.

3. Sprinkle the salmon with salt and grill 3 to 4 minutes per side, or until opaque throughout. Let stand 5 minutes. Cut salmon lengthwise into thin slices.

4. Place 1 nori sheet, shiny side down, on a sushi mat, covered with plastic wrap, with the long end toward you. Pat 1 cup rice mixture evenly over the nori with moist hands, leaving a 1-inch border on one long end of the nori. Arrange a few salmon slices, 2 stalks of asparagus, a few slices of avocado, and a few slices of red pepper along the bottom third of rice-covered nori. Spoon one-sixth of the wasabi along the length of the roll.

5. Lift the edge of the nori closest to you; fold it over the filling. Lift the bottom edge of the sushi mat; roll toward the top edge, pressing firmly on the sushi roll. Continue rolling to the top edge; press the mat to seal the sushi roll. Let rest, seam side down, for 5 minutes. Slice crosswise into 8 pieces. Repeat the procedure with the remaining nori, rice mixture, salmon, asparagus, avocado, red pepper, and wasabi.

Yield: 6 8-piece servings

Calories: 341; protein: 14 g; carbohydrate: 60 g; fiber: 6 g; sodium: 374 mg; fat: 7 g (saturated: 1.2 g; monounsaturated: 3.1 g; polyunsaturated: 2.2 g; trans: 0 g); cholesterol: 24 mg; folate: 41 mcg; iron: 2 mg

Orange-Glazed Salmon

Fatty fish like salmon are rich in omega-3 fatty acids, fats that are good for the heart and brain. They're also important for the developing fetus.

¼ teaspoon salt

4 6-ounce boneless, skinless salmon fillets

1 tablespoon orange marmalade

½ tablespoon rice wine vinegar

½ tablespoon orange juice concentrate

½ tablespoon soy sauce

1 teaspoon honey

2 teaspoons toasted sesame oil, divided

½ teaspoon chili garlic sauce

¼ teaspoon freshly grated ginger

1 tablespoon toasted sesame seeds

1. Sprinkle the salt on the fish.

2. Combine the marmalade, vinegar, orange juice concentrate, soy sauce, honey, 1 teaspoon of the sesame oil, chili sauce, and ginger in a shallow baking dish; whisk to blend. Add the salmon to the dish; cover and let marinate at room temperature for 30 minutes, turning once halfway through the marinating time.

3. Preheat the oven to 400°F.

4. Lightly coat an ovenproof nonstick skillet with the remaining 1 teaspoon of sesame oil and heat over medium heat. Add the fish to the pan and cook 3 to 4 minutes, or until lightly browned. Turn the fish

over and sprinkle with sesame seeds. Place the skillet in the oven; bake 6 to 8 minutes, or until the fish is opaque throughout.

Yield: 4 1-fillet servings

Calories: 334; protein: 40 g; carbohydrate: 6 g; fiber: 0 g; sodium: 376 mg; fat: 16 g (saturated: 2.3 g; monounsaturated: 5 g; polyunsaturated: 5.9 g; trans: 0 g); cholesterol: 107 mg; folate: 48 mcg; iron: 5 mg

Pecan-Crusted Tilapia with Mango Salsa

If you can't find tilapia (a mild-flavored farm-raised fish), substitute any mild white fish, like orange roughy, perch, or snapper. Mangos contain small amounts of folate.

    1 mango, peeled and diced
    2 tablespoons finely chopped red onion
    3 tablespoons chopped parsley, divided
    1 tablespoon fresh lime juice
    ½ cup pecan halves or pieces
    3 tablespoons fresh whole-grain bread crumbs
    ½ teaspoon salt, divided
    1 egg, lightly beaten
    ½ teaspoon water
    4 6-ounce tilapia fillets
    1 tablespoon olive or canola oil

1. Combine the mango, the onion, 2 tablespoons of the parsley, and the lime juice in a small bowl. Set aside.

2. Place the pecan halves, the bread crumbs, and ¼ teaspoon of the salt in a minichopper or blender and pulse until finely chopped. Place the mixture into a shallow bowl.

3. Combine the egg and ½ teaspoon of water in a separate shallow bowl.

4. Sprinkle the remaining ¼ teaspoon of salt on the fish; dip it into the egg mixture and then dredge it in the nut mixture, lightly coating both sides.

5. Heat the oil in a large nonstick skillet over medium heat. Add the fish and cook for 2 to 3 minutes, or until lightly browned. Flip and cook on the remaining side for 2 minutes, or until lightly browned.

Watch carefully so that the nuts do not burn; reduce the heat to medium low if necessary to prevent overcooking nuts.

6. To serve, place the fish on a platter and scatter the mango salsa over the top.

Yield: 4 servings of 1 fillet and ⅓ cup salsa

Calories: 303; protein: 28 g; carbohydrate: 12 g; fiber: 2 g; sodium: 431 mg; fat: 16 g (saturated: 1.8 g; monounsaturated: 9.6 g; polyunsaturated: 3.6 g; trans: 0 g); cholesterol: 87 mg; folate: 37 mcg; iron: 1 mg

Chili-Spiced Shrimp

To save time, look for fresh or frozen raw shrimp that are already peeled and deveined. If you prefer, leave the tails attached so the shrimp are easier to handle. Serve as an appetizer or toss with whole wheat fettuccini and olive oil for a main dish.

1 teaspoon chili powder

½ teaspoon minced dried onion flakes

½ teaspoon dried oregano

½ teaspoon sugar

½ teaspoon salt

¼ teaspoon crushed red pepper flakes

1¼ pounds medium shrimp, peeled and deveined

1 tablespoon olive or canola oil

1 teaspoon finely minced garlic

½ to 1 teaspoon seeded, finely minced jalapeño pepper

1. Combine the chili powder, onion flakes, oregano, sugar, salt, and red pepper flakes in a large bowl; stir to mix. Add the shrimp to the bowl and toss gently, so the shrimp are evenly coated with the spice mix.

2. Heat a large nonstick skillet over medium heat. Add the oil and heat. Stir in the garlic and jalapeño and cook for 30 seconds. Add the shrimp; sauté for 4 to 5 minutes, turning once halfway through the cooking time, until the shrimp are opaque.

Yield: 4 10-shrimp servings

Calories: 167; protein: 29 g; carbohydrate: 3 g; fiber: 0 g; sodium: 512 mg; fat: 4 g (saturated: 0.6 g; monounsaturated: 1.2 g; polyunsaturated: 1.1 g; trans: 0 g); cholesterol: 215 mg; folate: 6 mcg; iron: 4 mg

Asian Salmon Burgers

Serve these burgers with steamed baby bok choy and brown basmati rice. Or place them on a toasted whole-grain sesame seed bun and top with a dollop of mayonnaise enhanced with a little finely grated lemon zest.

1 ¼ pounds skinless, boneless salmon fillet, coarsely chopped
½ cup thinly sliced green onion
¼ cup fresh cilantro leaves
2 teaspoons peeled, minced fresh ginger
1 teaspoon chili garlic sauce
¾ teaspoon salt
¼ cup panko (Japanese bread crumbs) or fresh whole-grain bread crumbs
1 tablespoon olive or canola oil

1. Place the salmon, onion, cilantro, ginger, garlic sauce, and salt in a food processor and pulse until well blended. Alternately, finely dice the salmon and mix with the onion, cilantro, ginger, garlic sauce, and salt. Place the mixture into a small bowl; cover and refrigerate for 30 minutes to allow flavors to blend.

2. Shape the salmon mixture into 4 burger-shaped patties and flatten to ½ inch thick. Sprinkle the panko on both sides of the patties and press gently with your fingers to make the bread crumbs stick.

3. Heat the oil in a large nonstick skillet over medium heat. Add the patties and cook for 2 minutes, or until nicely browned. Flip and cook for 2 to 3 minutes, or until the fish is opaque throughout.

Yield: 4 1-burger servings

Calories: 286; protein: 33 g; carbohydrate: 5 g; fiber: 1 g; sodium: 612 mg; fat: 14 g (saturated: 2.1 g; monounsaturated: 5.9 g; polyunsaturated: 4.5 g; trans: 0 g); cholesterol: 90 mg; folate: 45 mcg; iron: 2 mg

Black Olive Pilaf with Roasted Vegetables

Asparagus, a good source of folate, is one of those vegetables that's enhanced by roasting. If you can't find whole wheat couscous, substitute fine- or medium-grain bulgur. But be sure to adjust and increase the cooking liquid based on package instructions.

1 pound asparagus, trimmed and cut into thirds

1 14-ounce can quartered artichoke hearts, drained and patted dry

1 cup julienned yellow and orange bell pepper

½ red onion, vertically sliced

3 tablespoons extra-virgin olive oil, divided

⅜ teaspoon salt, divided

1½ cups vegetable broth or water

½ teaspoon finely grated lemon zest

2 tablespoons lemon juice

1 7.6-ounce box whole wheat couscous (about 1⅓ cups)

½ cup shredded Parmesan cheese (2 ounces)

⅓ cup chopped black olives

¼ cup chopped basil or parsley

¼ teaspoon freshly ground black pepper

Fresh basil or parsley (optional)

1. Preheat the oven to 425°F.

2. Combine the asparagus, artichoke hearts, bell pepper, and onion in a bowl. Drizzle with 2 tablespoons of the oil. Toss gently to mix and place on a baking sheet lined with foil. Roast at 425°F for 22 to 25 minutes, or until the vegetables begin to brown lightly.

3. Turn off the oven. Sprinkle ¼ teaspoon salt on the vegetables and bring the ends of the foil together to wrap package style. Leave in the oven to keep warm.

4. Combine the broth, zest, juice, and remaining 1 tablespoon of oil and ⅛ teaspoon of salt in a small saucepan. Bring to a boil. Stir in

the couscous. Cover and remove from heat; let stand 5 minutes. Uncover; fluff the couscous with a fork. Stir in the cheese, olives, basil, and pepper.

5. To serve, spoon one-fourth of the couscous mixture onto each of 4 dinner plates. Top with vegetables. Garnish with fresh basil or parsley, if desired.

Yield: 4 servings of 1 cup couscous and 2/3 cup roasted vegetables

Calories: 389; protein: 15 g; carbohydrate: 55 g; fiber: 11 g; sodium: 664 mg; fat: 14 g (saturated: 3.2 g; monounsaturated: 8.5 g; polyunsaturated: 1.1 g; trans: 0 g); cholesterol: 7 mg; folate: 70 mcg; iron: 5 mg

Poblano and Black Bean Chili

This vegetarian chili delivers a good dose of iron and folate (the beans). And that iron is absorbed more easily because the dish also contains plenty of vitamin C from the bell peppers and tomatoes. If you're not a fan of hot, spicy food, try substituting milder Anaheim peppers for the poblano.

1 small poblano pepper, cut in half lengthwise and seeded
2 tablespoons olive oil
2 cups chopped onion
½ cup finely chopped celery
1 tablespoon chili powder
2 teaspoons cumin seeds, crushed
2 teaspoons dried oregano
1 teaspoon ground cumin
¾ teaspoon salt, divided
2 cups chopped assorted red, yellow, and orange bell peppers
2 14.5-ounce cans diced tomatoes
1 14.5-ounce can no-salt-added diced tomatoes
2 15-ounce cans black beans, drained
¼ cup finely chopped cilantro
Queso asadero cheese, crumbled (optional)

1. Preheat the broiler.

2. Flatten the poblano chili halves with your hands and place on a baking sheet lined with foil. Broil, 4 to 6 inches from heat, until the skins begin to blacken, about 5 to 7 minutes. Turn off the oven; pull the ends of the foil together and wrap the peppers tightly shut. Let stand 15 minutes, or until the skins loosen. Peel the skins and discard; finely chop the pepper.

3. Heat the oil in a large stockpot over medium heat. Add the onion and celery and cook for 6 to 8 minutes, or until the vegetables soften. Stir in the chili powder, the cumin seed, the oregano, the

ground cumin, and ½ teaspoon of the salt; cook for 1 minute. Add the bell peppers and tomatoes and bring to a boil; reduce heat, cover, and simmer for 10 minutes.

4. Uncover; stir in the beans, the remaining ¼ teaspoon of salt, and half of the roasted poblanos and cilantro and cook for 3 to 4 minutes, or until heated through. Taste for heat; add the remaining half of the poblanos, if desired.

5. To serve, spoon the chili into bowls. Sprinkle with cheese, if desired.

Yield: 9 1½-cup (without cheese) servings

Calories: 206; protein: 9 g; carbohydrate: 39 g; fiber: 13 g; sodium: 755 mg; fat: 5 g (saturated: 0.7 g; monounsaturated: 3.5 g; polyunsaturated: 0.7 g; trans: 0 g); cholesterol: 0 mg; folate: 24 mcg; iron: 4 mg

Notes

Chapter 1 Nourishing the Miracle of Conception

1. *Infertility: An Overview*. American Society for Reproductive Medicine. http://www.asrm.org/Patients/patientbooklets/ infertility_overview.pdf accessed on 14 July 2007.
2. Smoking and infertility. *Fertility and Sterility* 2006; 86:S172–177.
3. Multiple pregnancy associated with infertility therapy. *Fertility and Sterility* 2006; 86 Suppl 5:S106–110.
4. Missmer SA, Willet WC, and Hankinson SE, for the Nurses' Health Study Research Group. Dietary fat and the incidence of endometriosis. *American Journal of Epidemiology* 2007; 165 (Suppl):S24.
5. Morrison JA, Glueck CJ, and Wang P. Dietary trans fatty acid intake is associated with increased fetal loss. *Fertility and Sterility* 2008; 90:385–390.
6. Norman RJ. Presentation to the American Society of Reproductive Medicine, November 10, 2008, San Francisco.
7. Pal L, Shu J, Zeitlian G, and Hickmon C. Vitamin D insufficiency in reproductive years may be contributory to ovulatory infertility and PCOS. *Fertility and Sterility*, 2008; 90 (Suppl 1):Abstract O-38.

Chapter 2 Missed Conceptions

1. Morice P, Josset P, Chapron C, and Dubuisson JB. History of infertility. *Human Reproduction Update* 1995; 1:497–504.
2. Freedman DH. The aggressive egg. *Discover* 1992; 13:60–66.
3. Ehrmann DA. Polycystic ovary syndrome. *New England Journal of Medicine* 2005; 352:1223–36.
4. Marsh K and Brand-Miller J. The optimal diet for women with polycystic ovary syndrome? *British Journal of Nutrition* 2005; 94:154–165.
5. Wilcox AJ, Weinberg CR, and Baird DD. Timing of sexual intercourse in relation to ovulation. Effects on the probability of conception, survival of the pregnancy, and sex of the baby. *New England Journal of Medicine* 1995; 333:1517–21.

6. Smoking and infertility. American Society for Reproductive Medicine. http://www.asrm.org/Patients/FactSheets/smoking.pdf accessed on 14 July 2007.

7. Barbieri RL, Domar AD, and Loughlin KR. *Six Steps to Increased Fertility: An Integrated Medical and Mind/Body Program to Promote Conception.* New York: Simon & Schuster, 2000.

Chapter 3 A Diet for All Ages

1. U.S. Department of Agriculture, U.S. Department of Health and Human Services. Dietary Guidelines for Americans 2005. Washington, DC, 2005. http://www.healthierus.gov/dietaryguidelines accessed on 14 July 2007.

2. Willett WC, with Skerrett PJ. *Eat, Drink, and Be Healthy: The Harvard Medical School Guide to Healthy Eating.* New York: Free Press, 2005.

Chapter 4 Slow Carbs, Not Low Carbs

1. Zhang C, Liu S, Solomon CG, and Hu FB. Dietary fiber intake, dietary glycemic load, and the risk for gestational diabetes mellitus. *Diabetes Care* 2006; 29:2223–30.

2. Hjollund NH, Jensen TK, Bonde JP, Henriksen TB, Andersson AM, and Skakkebaek NE. Is glycosylated haemoglobin a marker of fertility? A follow-up study of first-pregnancy planners. *Human Reproduction* 1999; 14:1478–82.

3. Chavarro JE, Rich-Edwards JW, Rosner B, and Willett WC. A prospective study of dietary carbohydrate quantity and quality in relation to risk of ovulatory infertility. *European Journal of Clinical Nutrition* 2007; In press.

4. Trends in intake of energy and macronutrients—United States, 1971–2000. *MMWR Morbidity and Mortality Weekly Report* 2004; 53:80–82.

5. Foster-Powell K, Holt SH, and Brand-Miller JC. International table of glycemic index and glycemic load values: 2002. *American Journal of Clinical Nutrition* 2002; 76:5–56.

Chapter 5 Balancing Fats

1. Page IH, Stare FJ, Corcoran AC, Pollack H, and Wilkinson CF. Atherosclerosis and the fat content of the diet. *Journal of the American Medical Association* 1957; 164:2048–51.

2. Chavarro JE, Rich-Edwards JW, Rosner BA, and Willett WC. Dietary fatty acid intakes and the risk of ovulatory infertility. *American Journal of Clinical Nutrition* 2007; 85:231–237.

3. Allison DB, Egan SK, Barraj LM, Caughman C, Infante M, and Heimbach JT. Estimated intakes of trans fatty and other fatty

acids in the U.S. population. *Journal of the American Dietetic Association* 1999; 99:166–174.

4. Hibbeln JR, Davis JM, Steer C, Emmett P, Rogers I, Williams C, and Golding J. Maternal seafood consumption in pregnancy and neurodevelopmental outcomes in childhood (ALSPAC study): An observational cohort study. *Lancet* 2007; 369:578–585.

5. Mozaffarian D, Katan MB, Ascherio A, Stampfer MJ, and Willett WC. Trans fatty acids and cardiovascular disease. *New England Journal of Medicine* 2006; 354:1601–13.

6. Letter Report on Dietary Reference Intakes for Trans Fatty Acids. Institute of Medicine. http://www.iom.edu/Object.File/Master/13/083/TransFattyAcids.pdf accessed on 14 July 2007.

7. U.S. Department of Agriculture, U.S. Department of Health and Human Services. Dietary Guidelines for Americans 2005. Washington, DC, 2005. http://www.healthierus.gov/dietaryguidelines accessed on 14 July 2007.

8. Food Labeling: Trans Fatty Acids in Nutrition Labeling. Government Publishing Office. http://www.cfsan.fda.gov/~lrd/fr03711a.html accessed on 14 July 2007.

Chapter 6 Plant Protein Rules

1. Chavarro JE, Rich-Edwards JW, Rosner B, and Willett WC. Protein intake and ovulatory infertility. *American Journal of Obstetrics and Gynecology* 2007; In press.

2. Hu FB, Stampfer MJ, Manson JE, Rimm E, Colditz GA, Speizer FE, Hennekens CH, and Willett WC. Dietary protein and risk of ischemic heart disease in women. *American Journal of Clinical Nutrition* 1999; 70:221–227.

3. Kelemen LE, Kushi LH, Jacobs DR Jr, and Cerhan JR. Associations of dietary protein with disease and mortality in a prospective study of postmenopausal women. *American Journal of Epidemiology* 2005; 161:239–249.

4. Fung TT, Schulze M, Manson JE, Willett WC, and Hu FB. Dietary patterns, meat intake, and the risk of type 2 diabetes in women. *Archives of Internal Medicine* 2004; 164:2235–40.

5. Jiang R, Manson JE, Stampfer MJ, Liu S, Willett WC, and Hu FB. Nut and peanut butter consumption and risk of type 2 diabetes in women. *Journal of the American Medical Association* 2002; 288:2554–60.

6. van Dam RM, Willett WC, Rimm EB, Stampfer MJ, and Hu FB. Dietary fat and meat intake in relation to risk of type 2 diabetes in men. *Diabetes Care* 2002; 25:417–424.

7. Newberne PM and Rogers AE. The role of nutrients in cancer causation. *Princess Takamatsu Symposia* 1985; 16:205–222.

8. Halton TL and Hu FB. The effects of high protein diets on thermogenesis, satiety and weight loss: A critical review. *Journal of the American College of Nutrition* 2004; 23:373–385.

9. Eisenstein J, Roberts SB, Dallal G, and Saltzman E. High-protein weight-loss diets: Are they safe and do they work? A review of the experimental and epidemiologic data. *Nutrition Reviews* 2002; 60:189–200.

10. Gardner CD, Kiazand A, Alhassan S, Kim S, Stafford RS, Balise RR, Kraemer HC, and King AC. Comparison of the Atkins, Zone, Ornish, and LEARN diets for change in weight and related risk factors among overweight premenopausal women: The A to Z weight loss study: A randomized trial. *Journal of the American Medical Association* 2007; 297:969–977.

11. Brower M and Leon W. Union of Concerned Scientists. *The Consumer's Guide to Effective Environmental Choices: Practical Advice from the Union of Concerned Scientists.* New York: Three Rivers Press, 1999.

12. Steinfeld H, Gerber P, Wassenaar T, Castel V, Rosales M, and de Haan C. *Livestock's Long Shadow.* Rome: Food and Agriculture Organization, 2006.

13. Mozaffarian D and Rimm EB. Fish intake, contaminants, and human health: Evaluating the risks and the benefits. *Journal of the American Medical Association* 2006; 296:1885–99.

14. Institute of Medicine. *Seafood choices: Balancing benefits and risks.* Washington, DC: National Academies Press, 2007.

15. Hibbeln JR, Davis JM, Steer C, Emmett P, Rogers I, Williams C, and Golding J. Maternal seafood consumption in pregnancy and neurodevelopmental outcomes in childhood (ALSPAC study): An observational cohort study. *Lancet* 2007; 369:578–585.

Chapter 7 Take a Break, Skim

1. Cramer DW, Xu H, and Sahi T. Adult hypolactasia, milk consumption, and age-specific fertility. *American Journal of Epidemiology* 1994; 139:282–289.

2. Greenlee AR, Arbuckle TE, and Chyou PH. Risk factors for female infertility in an agricultural region. *Epidemiology* 2003; 14:429–436.

3. Chavarro JE, Rich-Edwards JW, Rosner B, and Willett WC. A prospective study of dairy foods intake and anovulatory infertility. *Human Reproduction* 2007; 22:1340–47.

4. FDA announces name changes for lower-fat milks and folic acid fortification for bakery products. Food and Drug Administration. http://www.cfsan.fda.gov/~lrd/hhmlkfol.html accessed on 14 July 2007.

5. Jenness R. Composition of milk. In: Wong NP, Jenness R, Kenney M, and Marth EH, eds. *Fundamentals of Dairy Chemistry.* New York: Van Nostrand Reinhold Co., 1988:19.

6. Adebamowo CA, Spiegelman D, Danby FW, Frazier AL, Willett WC, and Holmes MD. High school dietary dairy intake and teenage acne. *Journal of the American Academy of Dermatology* 2005; 52:207–214.

7. *The Changing Landscape of U.S. Milk Production.* USDA Economic Research Service. http://www.ers.usda.gov/publications/sb978/ sb978.pdf accessed on 14 July 2007.

8. got milk? gallery. National Milk Mustache "got milk?" campaign. http://www.milknewsroom.com/ads.htm accessed on 14 July 2007.

9. Fast facts on osteoporosis. National Osteoporosis Foundation. http://www.nof.org/osteoporosis/diseasefacts.htm accessed on 14 July 2007.

10. Lactose intolerance. National Institute of Diabetes and Digestive and Kidney Diseases. http://digestive.niddk.nih.gov/ddiseases/pubs/ lactoseintolerance/ accessed on 14 July 2007.

11. Calcium content of selected foods (sorted by nutrient content). USDA National Nutrient Database for Standard Reference, Release 18. http://www.nal.usda.gov/fnic/foodcomp/Data/SR18/nutrlist/ sr18w301.pdf accessed on 14 July 2007.

Chapter 8 Mighty Micros

1. National Institutes of Health state-of-the-science conference statement: Multivitamin/mineral supplements and chronic disease prevention. *Annals of Internal Medicine* 2006; 145:364–371.

2. Czeizel AE and Dudas I. Prevention of the first occurrence of neural-tube defects by periconceptional vitamin supplementation. *New England Journal of Medicine* 1992; 327:1832–35.

3. Czeizel AE, Dudas I, and Metneki J. Pregnancy outcomes in a randomised controlled trial of periconceptional multivitamin supplementation. Final report. *Archives of Gynecology and Obstetrics* 1994; 255:131–139.

4. Dudas I, Rockenbauer M, and Czeizel AE. The effect of preconceptional multivitamin supplementation on the menstrual cycle. *Archives of Gynecology and Obstetrics* 1995; 256:115–123.

5. Czeizel AE and Vargha P. Periconceptional folic acid/multivitamin supplementation and twin pregnancy. *American Journal of Obstetrics and Gynecology* 2004; 191:790–794.

6. Ericson A, Kallen B, and Aberg A. Use of multivitamins and folic acid in early pregnancy and multiple births in Sweden. *Twin Research* 2001; 4:63–66.

7. Waller DK, Tita AT, and Annegers JF. Rates of twinning before and after fortification of foods in the US with folic acid, Texas, 1996 to 1998. *Paediatric and Perinatal Epidemiology* 2003; 17:378–383.

8. Werler MM, Cragan JD, Wasserman CR, Shaw GM, Erickson JD, and Mitchell AA. Multivitamin supplementation and multiple births. *American Journal of Medical Genetics* 1997; 71:93–96.

9. Westphal LM, Polan ML, Trant AS, and Mooney SB. A nutritional supplement for improving fertility in women: A pilot study. *Journal of Reproductive Medicine* 2004; 49:289–293.

10. Chavarro JE, Rich-Edwards JW, Rosner BA, and Willett WC. Use of multivitamins, intake of B vitamins, and risk of ovulatory infertility: A prospective cohort study. *Fertility and Sterility*, 9 July 2007, doi: 10.1016/j-fertnstert.2007.03.089.

11. Chavarro JE, Rich-Edwards JW, Rosner BA, and Willett WC. Iron intake and risk of ovulatory infertility. *Obstetrics and Gynecology* 2006; 108:1145–52.

12. Hirson C. Coeliac infertility-folic-acid therapy. *Lancet* 1970; 1:412.

13. Dawson DW and Sawers AH. Infertility and folate deficiency. Case reports. *British Journal of Obstetrics and Gynaecology* 1982; 89:678–680.

14. Harper AF, Lindemann MD, Chiba LI, Combs GE, Handlin DL, Kornegay ET, and Southern LL. An assessment of dietary folic acid levels during gestation and lactation on reproductive and lactational performance of sows: A cooperative study. S-145 Committee on Nutritional Systems for Swine to Increase Reproductive Efficiency. *Journal of Animal Science* 1994; 72:2338–44.

15. Thaler CJ, Budiman H, Ruebsamen H, Nagel D, and Lohse P. Effects of the common 677C>T mutation of the 5, 10-methylenetetrahydrofolate reductase (MTHFR) gene on ovarian responsiveness to recombinant follicle-stimulating hormone. *American Journal of Reproductive Immunology* 2006; 55:251–258.

16. Folate intake by women of child-bearing age: The impact of fortification. U.S. Department of Agriculture. http://www.cnpp.usda.gov/Publications/NutritionInsights/Insight30.pdf accessed on 14 July 2007.

17. Folate status in women of childbearing age, by race/ethnicity— United States, 1999–2000, 2001–2002, and 2003–2004. *MMWR Morbidity and Mortality Weekly Report* 2007; 55:1377–80.

18. Iron deficiency—United States, 1999–2000. *MMWR Morbidity and Mortality Weekly Report* 2002; 51:897–899.

19. Goh YI, Bollano E, Einarson TR, and Koren G. Prenatal multivitamin supplementation and rates of congenital anomalies: A meta-analysis. *Journal of Obstetrics and Gynaecology Canada* 2006; 28:680–689.

20. Wilcox AJ, Lie RT, Solvoll K, Taylor J, McConnaughey DR, Abyholm F, Vindenes H, Vollset SE, and Drevon CA. Folic acid supplements and risk of facial clefts: National population based case-control study. *British Medical Journal.* 2007; 334: 464–467.

21. Bezold G, Lange M, and Peter RU. Homozygous methylenetetra-hydrofolate reductase C677T mutation and male infertility. *New England Journal of Medicine* 2001; 344:1172–73.

22. Lee HC, Jeong YM, Lee SH, Cha KY, Song SH, Kim NK, Lee KW, and Lee S. Association study of four polymorphisms in three folate-related enzyme genes with non-obstructive male infertility. *Human Reproduction* 2006; 21:3162–70.

23. Wong WY, Merkus HM, Thomas CM, Menkveld R, Zielhuis GA, and Steegers-Theunissen RP. Effects of folic acid and zinc sulfate on male factor subfertility: A double-blind, randomized, placebo-controlled trial. *Fertility and Sterility* 2002; 77:491–498.

24. Serdula MK, Gillespie C, Kettel-Khan L, Farris R, Seymour J, and Denny C. Trends in fruit and vegetable consumption among adults in the United States: Behavioral risk factor surveillance system, 1994–2000. *American Journal of Public Health* 2004; 94:1014–18.

Chapter 9 Drink (Water) to Your Health

1. Chavarro JE, Rich-Edwards JW, Rosner B, and Willett WC. Caffeinated and alcoholic beverage intake in relation to the risk of ovulatory disorder infertility. In preparation 2007.

2. Collins TFX, Welsh JJ, Black TN, and Collins EV. A study of the teratogenic potential of caffeine given by oral intubation to rats. *Regulatory Toxicology and Pharmacology* 1981; 1:355–378.

3. Collins TF, Welsh JJ, Black TN, and Ruggles DI. A study of the teratogenic potential of caffeine ingested in drinking-water. *Food and Chemical Toxicology* 1983; 21:763–777.

4. Hatch EE and Bracken MB. Association of delayed conception with caffeine consumption. *American Journal of Epidemiology* 1993; 138:1082–92.

5. Grodstein F, Goldman MB, Ryan L, and Cramer DW. Relation of female infertility to consumption of caffeinated beverages. *American Journal of Epidemiology* 1993; 137:1353–60.

6. Jensen TK, Henriksen TB, Hjollund NH, Scheike T, Kolstad H, Giwercman A, Ernst E, Bonde JP, Skakkebaek NE, and Olsen J. Caffeine intake and fecundability: A follow-up study among 430 Danish couples planning their first pregnancy. *Reproductive Toxicology* 1998; 12:289–295.

7. McCusker RR, Goldberger BA, and Cone EJ. Caffeine content of specialty coffees. *Journal of Analytical Toxicology* 2003; 27:520–522.

8. Caan B, Quesenberry CP Jr, and Coates AO. Differences in fertility associated with caffeinated beverage consumption. *American Journal of Public Health* 1998; 88:270–274.

9. Grodstein F, Goldman MB, and Cramer DW. Infertility in women and moderate alcohol use. *American Journal of Public Health* 1994; 84:1429–32.

10. Tolstrup JS, Kjaer SK, Holst C, Sharif H, Munk C, Osler M, Schmidt L, Andersen AM, and Gronbaek M. Alcohol use as predictor for infertility in a representative population of Danish women. *Acta Obstetricia et Gynecologica Scandinavica* 2003; 82:744–749.

11. Juhl M, Nybo Andersen AM, Gronbaek M, and Olsen J. Moderate alcohol consumption and waiting time to pregnancy. *Human Reproduction* 2001; 16:2705–09.

12. Juhl M, Olsen J, Nybo Andersen AM, and Gronbaek M. Intake of wine, beer and spirits and waiting time to pregnancy. *Human Reproduction* 2003; 18:1967–71.

13. Mukherjee RA, Hollins S, Abou-Saleh MT, and Turk J. Low level alcohol consumption and the fetus. *British Medical Journal* 2005; 330:375–376.

14. Emanuele MA and Emanuele NV. Alcohol's effects on male reproduction. *Alcohol Health and Research World* 1998; 22:195–201.

15. Henriksen TB, Hjollund NH, Jensen TK, Bonde JP, Andersson AM, Kolstad H, Ernst E, Giwercman A, Skakkebaek NE, and Olsen J. Alcohol consumption at the time of conception and spontaneous abortion. *American Journal of Epidemiology* 2004; 160:661–667.

16. Klonoff-Cohen H, Lam-Kruglick P, and Gonzalez C. Effects of maternal and paternal alcohol consumption on the success rates of in vitro fertilization and gamete intrafallopian transfer. *Fertility and Sterility* 2003; 79:330–339.

Chapter 10 The 7½ Percent Solution

1. Weight and fertility. American Society for Reproductive Medicine. http://www.asrm.org/Patients/FactSheets/weightfertility.pdf accessed on 14 July 2007.

2. *Clinical Guidelines on the Identification, Evaluation, and Treatment of Overweight and Obesity in Adults.* National Institutes of Health, National Heart, Lung, and Blood Institute, Obesity Education Initiative. http://www.nhlbi.nih.gov/guidelines/obesity/ob_gdlns.pdf accessed on 14 July 2007.

3. Stein Z and Susser M. Fertility, fecundity, famine: Food rations in the Dutch famine 1944/5 have a causal relation to fertility, and probably to fecundity. *Human Biology* 1975; 47:131–154.

4. Gosman GG, Katcher HI, and Legro RS. Obesity and the role of gut and adipose hormones in female reproduction. *Human Reproduction Update* 2006; 12:585–601.

5. Rich-Edwards JW, Spiegelman D, Garland M, Hertzmark E, Hunter DJ, Colditz GA, Willett WC, Wand H, and Manson JE. Physical activity, body mass index, and ovulatory disorder infertility. *Epidemiology* 2002; 13:184–190.

6. Ratner R, Goldberg R, Haffner S, Marcovina S, Orchard T, Fowler S, and Temprosa M. Impact of intensive lifestyle and metformin therapy on cardiovascular disease risk factors in the diabetes prevention program. *Diabetes Care* 2005; 28:888–894.

7. McManus K, Antinoro L, and Sacks F. A randomized controlled trial of a moderate-fat, low-energy diet compared with a low-fat, low-energy diet for weight loss in overweight adults. *International Journal of Obesity and Related Metabolic Disorders* 2001; 25:1503–11.

8. Dansinger ML, Gleason JA, Griffith JL, Selker HP, and Schaefer EJ. Comparison of the Atkins, Ornish, Weight Watchers, and Zone diets for weight loss and heart disease risk reduction: A randomized trial. *Journal of the American Medical Association* 2005; 293:43–53.

9. Gardner CD, Kiazand A, Alhassan S, Kim S, Stafford RS, Balise RR, Kraemer HC, and King AC. Comparison of the Atkins, Zone, Ornish, and LEARN diets for change in weight and related risk factors among overweight premenopausal women: The A to Z weight loss study: A randomized trial. *Journal of the American Medical Association* 2007; 297:969–977.

10. DiMeglio DP, and Mattes RD. Liquid versus solid carbohydrate: Effects on food intake and body weight. *International Journal of Obesity and Related Metabolic Disorders* 2000; 24:794–800.

11. Sallmen M, Sandler DP, Hoppin JA, Blair A, and Baird DD. Reduced fertility among overweight and obese men. *Epidemiology* 2006; 17:520–523.

Chapter 11 You've Got to Move It, Move It

1. Saltin B, Blomqvist G, Mitchell JH, Johnson RL Jr, Wildenthal K, and Chapman CB. Response to exercise after bed rest and after training. *Circulation* 1968; 38 (5 Suppl):VII1–VII78.

2. McGuire DK, Levine BD, Williamson JW, Snell PG, Blomqvist CG, Saltin B, and Mitchell JH. A 30-year follow-up of the Dallas Bedrest and Training Study. *Circulation* 2001; 104:1350–66.

3. Kortebein P, Ferrando A, Lombeida J, Wolfe R, and Evans WJ. Effect of 10 days of bed rest on skeletal muscle in healthy older adults. *Journal of the American Medical Association* 2007; 297:1772–74.

4. *Physical Activity and Health: A Report of the Surgeon General.* U.S. Department of Health and Human Services, Centers for Disease Control and Prevention. http://www.cdc.gov/nccdphp/sgr/sgr.htm accessed on 14 July 2007.

5. Frisch RE. *Female Fertility and the Body Fat Connection.* Chicago: University of Chicago Press, 2002.

6. Bullen BA, Skrinar GS, Beitins IZ, von Mering G, Turnbull BA, and McArthur JW. Induction of menstrual disorders by strenuous exercise in untrained women. *New England Journal of Medicine* 1985; 312:1349–53.

7. Stein Z and Susser M. Fertility, fecundity, famine: Food rations in the Dutch famine 1944/5 have a causal relation to fertility, and probably to fecundity. *Human Biology* 1975; 47:131–154.

8. Prentice AM, Rayco-Solon P, and Moore SE. Insights from the developing world: Thrifty genotypes and thrifty phenotypes. *Proceedings of the Nutrition Society* 2005; 64:153–161.

9. Rich-Edwards JW, Spiegelman D, Garland M, Hertzmark E, Hunter DJ, Colditz GA, Willett WC, Wand H, and Manson JE. Physical activity, body mass index, and ovulatory disorder infertility. *Epidemiology* 2002; 13:184–190.

10. Simon HB. *The No Sweat Exercise Plan: Lose Weight, Get Healthy, and Live Longer.* New York: McGraw-Hill, 2006.

11. Institute of Medicine. *Dietary Reference Intakes for Energy, Carbohydrate, Fiber, Fat, Fatty Acids, Cholesterol, Protein, and Amino Acids (Macronutrients).* Washington, DC: National Academies Press, 2002.

12. Zeni AI, Hoffman MD, and Clifford PS. Energy expenditure with indoor exercise machines. *Journal of the American Medical Association* 1996; 275:1424–27.

13. Wallace JP, Raglin JS, and Jastremski CA. Twelve month adherence of adults who joined a fitness program with a spouse vs. without a spouse. *Journal of Sports Medicine and Physical Fitness* 1995; 35:206–213.

14. Cordain L, Gotshall RW, Eaton SB, and Eaton SB, 3rd. Physical activity, energy expenditure and fitness: An evolutionary perspective. *International Journal of Sports Medicine* 1998; 19:328–335.

Chapter 12 Putting It All Together

1. Chavarro JE, Rich-Edwards JW, Rosner B, and Willett WC. Diet and lifestyle in the prevention of ovulatory disorder infertility. *Obstetrics and Gynecology* 2007; In press.

Index